POLIO

POLIO

Daniel J. Wilson

Biographies of Disease
Julie K. Silver, M.D., Series Editor

GREENWOOD PRESS
An Imprint of ABC-CLIO, LLC

A B C 🔖 C L I O

Santa Barbara, California • Denver, Colorado • Oxford, England

Library of Congress Cataloging-in-Publication Data

Wilson, Daniel J., 1949–
  Polio / Daniel J. Wilson.
    p. cm. — (Biographies of disease)
  Includes bibliographical references and index.
  ISBN 978-0-313-35897-5 (hard copy : alk. paper) — ISBN 978-0-313-35898-2
(e-book) 1. Poliomyelitis—Popular works. I. Title.
  RC180.2.W473 2009
  616.8'35—dc22   2009027933

13 12 11 10 9 1 2 3 4 5

This book is also available on the World Wide Web as an eBook.
Visit www.abc-clio.com for details.

ABC-CLIO, LLC
130 Cremona Drive, P.O. Box 1911
Santa Barbara, California 93116-1911

This book is printed on acid-free paper ∞

Manufactured in the United States of America

Contents

Series Foreword

Every disease has a story to tell: about how it started long ago and began to disable or even take the lives of its innocent victims, about the way it hurts us, and about how we are trying to stop it. In this Biographies of Disease series, the authors tell the stories of the diseases that we have come to know and dread. The stories of these diseases have all of the components that make for great literature. There is incredible drama played out in real-life scenes from the past, present, and future. You'll read about how men and women of science stumbled trying to save the lives of those they aimed to protect. Turn the pages and you'll also learn about the amazing success of those who fought for health and won, often saving thousands of lives in the process. If you don't want to be a health professional or research scientist now, when you finish this book you may think differently. The men and women in this book are heroes who often risked their own lives to save or improve ours. This is the biography of a disease, but it is also the story of real people who made incredible sacrifices to stop it in its tracks.

Julie K. Silver, M.D.
Assistant Professor, Harvard Medical School
Department of Physical Medicine and Rehabilitation

Acknowledgments

Although writing is a solitary occupation, no book is written without the support of others, and this book is no exception. I would like to thank Julie Silver, M.D., for suggesting that I write *Polio*, and for her support during the process. Her invitation gave me an opportunity to think seriously about how to present the history of polio to a wider audience.

I owe Muhlenberg College a debt of gratitude as well. The manuscript was written while I held the Class of 1932 Research Professorship, which provided a year without teaching. I also appreciate the support I received from President Randy Helm, Provost Margie Hass, Professor John Malsberger, chair of the history department, and my colleagues on the Faculty Development and Scholarship Committee. The librarians of Trexler Library were most helpful on several occasions in tracking down information.

I particularly want to thank David Rose, archivist of the March of Dimes, for his valuable assistance in choosing the images that appear in the book. I also want to thank the March of Dimes Foundation for permission to use the photographs and the cover image.

David Paige and the other editors and staff at ABC-CLIO/Greenwood were a pleasure to work with.

While writing this book, Chet DiRomualdo and his crew were remodeling part of the house. I want to thank him and his entire crew, but especially Ron, John, and Kevin, for providing a welcome distraction from the computer.

Friends and family once again supported my writing endeavors. I am thankful for the continuing support and encouragement of Melissa Barker, Dave and Sally Keehn, Louise and Carl Kempka, Kay Klausmeier, Dotty and George Kriebel, Judy and Alan Morrison, Paul and Beth Paskoff, Robert and Jennifer Scavuzzo, Bart and Diane Shaw, Larry Shiner, Bob Streich, Emily and Joseph Vincent, Marjorie Wilson, and Stewart Wilson.

Finally, my greatest debt, as always, is to my wife Carol, who provided wonderful support and encouragement in so many ways.

1

Poliomyelitis and the Poliovirus

September of 1955 was warm in northern Wisconsin, almost like summer. I was five and not yet in school. I remember feeling sick and lying on a cot we kept on our screened-in porch. When I didn't get better after a day or two, my mother phoned the family's doctor. In the 1950s physicians still made house calls to examine patients, and, before long, Dr. Freeman was beside my cot. He asked me to raise my head off the pillow, and I was unable. There was a worried look on his face, and he did a couple of other tests. Then, he and my parents had a whispered conversation. Soon after the doctor left, my parents informed me that I would be going to the hospital. My father picked me up in his strong arms and carried me to the car. It was a short ride to the hospital, where my father carried me in. At the hospital I began to cry when I realized that my parents were going to leave me there, as I had never been left anywhere alone before. A nurse picked me up and carried me to a crib. My parents were left outside the room, and I could only see them through the window in the door. I was still crying when they left. Later I learned that I had come down with polio, one of almost 29,000 cases diagnosed nationwide that year.

WHAT IS POLIO?

Polio was the most feared childhood disease of the first half of the twentieth century. During polio epidemics schools, movie theaters, and swimming pools were closed to prevent the spread of the disease. Parents kept their children inside in hopes that it would protect them from exposure to the poliovirus. In spite of all the precautions, every summer tens of thousands of children contracted the disease, became acutely sick, and were permanently paralyzed. When the poliovirus paralyzed the muscles that controlled breathing, the patient died unless his or her breathing was assisted by a large metal respirator known as an iron lung. As the century wore on, doctors realized that although most of their polio patients were children, adolescents and even adults could contract the disease. The best-known polio patient, in fact, was Franklin D. Roosevelt, an aspiring politician and future president of the United States, who developed polio in 1921 when he was 39.

The illness Americans know as polio has had several names since the middle of the nineteenth century, when it was recognized as a distinct disease. French doctors initially called the disease *infantile paralysis* because paralysis in young children was its most significant symptom. This became one of the common names for the disease in the twentieth century, even after it became known that teenagers and adults could contract the disease. Doctors eventually settled on the name *poliomyelitis*. Poliomyelitis is derived from several Greek words referring to the parts of the spinal cord where the poliovirus does its damage. The word means an inflammation of the gray marrow of the spinal cord. Although doctors continued to refer to the disease as poliomyelitis, most Americans in the middle of the twentieth century knew it simply as polio.

Polio is a viral disease caused by the poliovirus. Individuals infected with polio shed the virus in their fecal material. In conditions of poor sanitation where human waste gets into the water supply or contaminates the dirt children play in, the poliovirus is easily ingested. Once it is taken into the digestive tract, the poliovirus most often causes an intestinal flu accompanied by aches, pains, and a fever. In about 90 percent of cases the poliovirus simply stays within the intestinal tract. Doctors call this *inapparent polio* because the virus never gains a foothold in the spinal cord and causes no apparent illness. The children infected recover and are immune to that particular strain of polio because of the antibodies their body produced. In 4 to 8 percent of infections the poliovirus causes a minor illness that was often previously diagnosed as summer flu. Again, there is no paralysis in these cases and the antibodies produced protect the child from catching that strain of poliovirus again. In less than 5 percent of infections, and for reasons that are still not well understood, the poliovirus succeeds in getting into the central nervous system in the spinal cord and producing a severe illness. Here the virus does the damage that causes its characteristic paralysis.

Once the poliovirus enters the spinal cord of an infected individual it damages or destroys specialized nerve cells called *anterior horn cells*. These cells are a key link in the motor neuron system that transmits messages from the brain to the muscles telling them to contract or relax so that we can move. When these anterior horn cells are damaged or destroyed, the nerves serving a particular set of muscles cease to function and the muscle is paralyzed. The extent of the damage and destruction determines the extent of the paralysis. If the nerve cells are simply damaged, the paralysis may be temporary and the patient may over time regain most or all of his or her muscle function. When the nerves are destroyed by the poliovirus, the paralysis is permanent since nerve cells are unable to regenerate. If only a few nerve cells are destroyed, the patient may experience weakness in that muscle because many nerve cells service each of the major muscle systems in the body. Individuals whose spinal cords were invaded by the poliovirus but who show no or only very mild muscle weakness have what doctors call *abortive poliomyelitis*. However, if the destruction is extensive, that muscle will be permanently paralyzed, and the patient may lose the ability to move an arm or leg, or be unable to breathe. These individuals have a classic case of *paralytic poliomyelitis*.

A case of polio usually begins innocently enough. The child or young adult begins to feel ill with muscle aches and weakness, a headache, perhaps an upset stomach, and a fever. Many people went to bed at the beginning of their symptoms, which it was discovered was the best thing to do. There is some evidence that if individuals continued their normal activities after the onset of the illness the severity of the illness and the extent of paralysis were likely to be greater. However, some adolescents might have had a big game or concert coming up or some adults might have had work responsibilities, so they pushed on until they were no longer able.

As the illness progressed there were certain signs that parents and doctors both looked for and feared. A stiff neck and the inability to touch one's chin to one's chest were indicators of paralytic polio. Many young people discovered how serious their illness was when they got out of bed to go to the bathroom and collapsed on the floor because their leg muscles were too weak to hold them. For some, it was the last unaided walk they would ever take. Doctors were usually called when signs of paralysis began to appear. In the first part of the twentieth century, family physicians commonly made house calls. The doctor would confirm what the parents feared—their child had polio. An ambulance was then called to rush the patient to the hospital, or perhaps the parents drove the child to the hospital themselves. It was a scene repeated again and again during the polio epidemics of the first six decades of the twentieth century.

ENDEMIC VERSUS EPIDEMIC POLIO

Epidemic diseases are those that occur periodically when a disease-causing virus is introduced into a community lacking immunity to the disease. Epidemic diseases began to occur early in human history once humans began to live in settled agricultural communities. Some human diseases apparently were derived from animal diseases following the domestication of animals, at which time humans began to live in close proximity to their animals. Epidemic diseases can be spread through the air or contaminated water and food. Where human sanitation practices are primitive, water and food are easily contaminated. The higher population densities that agriculture made possible also contributed to the spread of epidemic diseases because the close living proximities allowed the diseases to be more easily passed among people.

Epidemic diseases often provide immunity to the individuals who survive, protecting them if they are exposed to the virus again later in life. Once an epidemic disease swept through a community and infected those without immunity, it often disappeared for a number of years since those who survived were immune. But many human epidemic diseases returned again and again to the same location. Some epidemic diseases, such as the plague, smallpox, and HIV/AIDS, have been major killers of humans. Although modern sanitation and modern medicine, particularly vaccines and antibiotics, have reduced the toll of epidemic disease, among these only smallpox has been eradicated.

Endemic diseases are those that are commonplace in a particular location. These diseases are almost always present, often year-around. They occur where environmental conditions permit the disease-causing organism to be continually present and able to infect humans. Some of these diseases may be acquired from contaminated water supplies, others by direct transmission from an infected individual, and others through the bite of an infected insect such as a mosquito. Some of these diseases can be quite serious and fatal, such as malaria and yellow fever in the tropical regions.

Polio had not always been an epidemic disease, one that thousands of individuals contracted over a short period of time. Historical evidence from Asia and Africa, where polio still exists, suggest that for much of history, polio was an endemic disease. That is, in situations where human sanitation is primitive the poliovirus circulates continually through the community. Most infants and children in these areas are exposed to the virus and infected when they are very young and still protected by antibodies that they acquired from their mothers. In this situation, children acquire their own antibodies to polio early on, when the disease is less likely to be paralytic. The older a person is when he or she is exposed to the poliovirus, the more likely the disease is to be paralytic. When polio is endemic, most children grow up protected from the virus and only a few children are paralyzed. However, in the nineteenth century, methods of disposing of human waste began to improve. Improvements in human sanitation, such as indoor toilets, sewers, and waste disposal plants, meant that the poliovirus was prevented from contaminating water supplies and soil. When this happened in Europe and the United States, children were no longer regularly exposed to the poliovirus and infected while protected by the maternal antibodies. Sanitary measures were never perfect, however, and at some point the poliovirus was again introduced to a community. Now, the older children, no longer protected by their mother's antibodies, became infected. These communities of unprotected older children would suddenly experience a significant number of paralytic cases in a short period of time.

Beginning in the late nineteenth century, doctors in both the United States and Europe began to recognize and describe small epidemics of polio. In the United States polio would remain an epidemic disease from the late 1800s until it was essentially eradicated by the polio vaccines in the 1960s.

2

Early Evidence of Polio and the First Epidemics

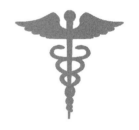

No one knows when the first case of polio occurred in humans. All the evidence suggests that polio has afflicted humans for a very long time, certainly from well before the time of written medical records. Polio probably emerged as a human disease sometime after men and women began to settle in villages, towns, and cities following the development of agriculture. But polio was unrecognized for many millennia because of several of its characteristics. Remember that over 90 percent of all infections are inapparent and that only about 3 to 5 percent of infections cause permanent paralysis. Remember, too, that in conditions of poor sanitation, such as existed through much of human history, polio becomes endemic in a population, continually circulating and infecting infants while they are still protected by maternal antibodies and before infections are likely to cause paralysis. Polio undoubtedly caused occasional paralysis in children during these many thousands of years, but given all the other maladies that affected humans until recently, an occasional paralyzed limb in a child did not seem particularly remarkable. With so many other causes of infant mortality, even an occasional death from polio easily escaped attention. Nonetheless, there is some evidence even from ancient times that polio existed in its paralytic form.

EARLY EVIDENCE OF POLIO

Historians, physicians, and archeologists have found evidence of what were likely cases of polio going as far back as the earliest records. While these records are not definitive proof that polio has long paralyzed humans, they describe the characteristic paralysis of the disease and provide the best evidence we are likely to get. One of the earliest descriptions is actually from an ancient Egyptian wall carving from the Eighteenth Dynasty (1580–1350 B.C.E.), or about 3,500 years ago. It shows a young man, perhaps a priest, with one withered leg and a drooping foot who supports himself with a staff. A leg paralyzed by polio usually withers because the muscles no longer work or build strength and size. Many modern polio patients suffered from drooping feet similar to that of the young man in the carving. While it is possible that another disease or an accident caused the young man's deformity, in the judgment of most experts who have viewed the image, polio is the most likely cause. That means polio has been infecting humans for at least 3,500 years.

The next suggestive evidence appears in written records from ancient Greece and Rome. The writings of the Greek physician Hippocrates (ca. 460 B.C.E.) contain descriptions of foot and leg deformities that might plausibly be describing paralytic polio. Several centuries later, the Roman physician Galen (138–201 C.E.) seems to have been familiar with paralysis of the legs that occurred in early childhood, again suggestive of polio. There is, of course, no way to prove that these were descriptions of polio, but the visual and textual evidence is tantalizing (Paul, 1971, pp. 14–15).

From the time of the ancient Rome to the eighteenth century, there is no clear evidence of polio in either the surviving written or visual evidence. There is, however, some evidence from this long time span that children and young adults continued to suffer from paralyzed limbs that would often produce grotesque deformities. From 200 to 1700 C.E., many visual artists seemed to delight in portraying deformed bodies, but whether any of these impairments were the result of polio is uncertain.

It is only in the 1700s that we again had descriptions of illnesses and paralysis that are suggestive of polio. There are a number of medical accounts from doctors in colonial America that describe sudden paralysis in young children affecting limbs on one side or another. Perhaps the clearest indication of polio comes from the illness that struck the Scottish author Walter Scott some eighteen months after his birth in Edinburgh in 1771. Healthy until this point, young Walter came down with a fever that seemed to be associated with the cutting of his teeth. The fever lasted three days, and on the fourth day when his parents bathed him they discovered that he was unable to move his right leg. The doctors who were consulted could offer no explanation for this puzzling paralysis. As he grew, Walter kept trying to use his leg and eventually he rebuilt its strength and learned to stand, walk, and run. That right leg, however, always remained smaller and weaker than his left one. In addition to this relatively detailed description of Scott's illness and paralysis, scattered throughout the medical literature of eighteenth-century England are other, briefer accounts of young children developing a fever that was followed a few days later by weakness, lameness, or paralysis (Paul, 1971, pp. 17–19).

FIRST MODERN MEDICAL DESCRIPTIONS OF POLIO

The first physician to give a modern clinical description of polio was the London pediatrician Michael Underwood, who published a book on the illnesses of children in 1784. There is no mention of a polio-like disease in the first edition of the book, but in the second edition (published in 1789) Underwood describes what he called "Debility of the Lower Extremities." The debility was lameness in the legs following the development of a fever. In subsequent editions of his medical text Underwood provided a fuller description of this disease. He described an illness that attacked infants and children and that weakened and paralyzed both arms and legs. Underwood also noted that some patients eventually regained strength in the affected limbs. During the early nineteenth century, additional clinical descriptions of what was probably polio appeared in medical literature in both Europe and the United States. One of the most fully developed descriptions came from Dr. Jacob von Heine, a German orthopedist, in a book published in 1840. Heine's book described fourteen cases in patients younger than three in which a disease with a fever was followed by paralysis of one or both legs. Heine suspected that the spinal cord was implicated in the paralysis, and he developed exercises, simple surgeries, and bracing to help his patients recover. Up to this point, no one, including Heine, recognized that this puzzling disease was contagious or had the potential to cause an epidemic (Paul, 1971, pp. 20–24, 30–33, 36).

Medical reports in Europe in the nineteenth century first reported clusters of fevers followed by paralysis in children. These clusters of what was probably polio occurred in central England in 1835, on the isolated South Atlantic island of St. Helena between 1830 and 1836, and in Louisiana in 1841. The Louisiana outbreak occurred in West Feliciana Parish. Dr. George Colmer noted that when he visited the community parents told him of eight to ten cases of children under two who had in the previous months suffered from paralysis in their limbs following a fever that developed while they were teething. Dr. Colmer also noted that all of the children had either recovered or were improving. These widely separated occurrences may have been the first recorded epidemics of polio, but there were probably others that went unrecognized and unrecorded (Paul, 1971, pp. 37–47).

With more frequent outbreaks occurring, scientists in Europe in the 1860s and 1870s also began to investigate the causes of this childhood paralysis. The great French neurologist Jean-Martin Charcot and his assistant A. Joffroy were the first scientists to demonstrate that the cause of paralysis was damage and destruction of the gray matter of the anterior horn cells of the spinal cord. When these cells were destroyed, they could no longer transmit motor impulses to the muscles, and paralysis resulted. These scientists had conducted an autopsy on a woman who had had polio as a child, and they described their findings in an article published in 1870 (Paul, 1971, pp. 54–57).

In the last third of the nineteenth century descriptions of polio proliferated and both clinical and laboratory knowledge of the disease expanded. In the United States, Dr. Mary Putnam Jacobi published a long article on polio in *A System of Medicine by American Authors* edited and published by Dr. William Pepper in 1886. Jacobi's article summarized the state of both clinical and scientific knowledge about polio based on her review of the European medical literature. She was also one of the first physicians in the United States to use the term "infantile paralysis" for the disease. This name would remain in common use down to the end of the epidemics in the 1950s (Paul, 1971, pp. 66–69).

FIRST MODERN AMERICAN EPIDEMIC

In the late 1880s and early 1890s, doctors began to notice an increasing number of polio cases, especially in and around Boston. There were, for example, twenty-six cases in eastern Massachusetts in the summer of 1893. The following year the first significant and well-documented epidemic of polio occurred in nearby Vermont. Dr. Charles S. Caverly, who was a public health officer for the state, provided the best description of the epidemic. It began in June in Rutland and Wallingford and by July had spread to other towns and villages in the state. Caverly's investigations revealed 132 cases of mainly infants and children. However, somewhat surprisingly, a number of adults were also diagnosed with the disease. Many patients recovered, but at least thirty were permanently paralyzed and 13.5 percent of the patients died. Since polio is more likely to be fatal among older patients, the relatively high death rate in the Vermont epidemic was not surprising (Paul, 1971, pp. 79–81).

In the years following the Vermont epidemic, polio continued to appear in the northeastern states. It is difficult to know just how widespread these cases of polio were because the doctors were not always required to report their diagnosis of the disease to public health authorities. In New York, for example, polio did not become a reportable disease until 1911. The largest outbreak in the first decade of the twentieth century occurred in New York in 1907, when there were over 1,000 cases in and around the city. Because the disease was not yet reportable, many mild cases probably went unrecognized by parents and unrecorded by physicians. The Vermont epidemic of 1894 and the New York epidemic of 1907 did suggest that the disease was beginning to change its character and its prevalence. Epidemics of polio were increasing in frequency, size, and severity. Although most polio patients were young children, the number of older children and even adults who succumbed to the disease was rising. The increasing number of older patients was particularly worrisome because it was more likely to be severe and paralytic among them.

NEW YORK EPIDEMIC OF 1916

In spite of the increasing occurrence of polio in the northeast, doctors, public health officials, and parents were unprepared for the size and severity of the 1916 epidemic in New York and surrounding states. The epidemic began in June and lasted until November. In that time there were over 27,000 cases reported in twenty-six states. There were approximately 6,000 deaths (22 percent of the total). New York City recorded over 8,900 cases and 2,400 deaths (27 percent of the cases) (Rogers, 1992, pp. 10–11). The epidemic frightened parents and children and strained the capacity of hospitals and the public health system.

During the first five months of 1916 public health officials had little reason to worry about polio. Only seventeen cases of the disease had been reported in the boroughs of the city. However, early June saw a worrisome increase in polio cases, especially in Brooklyn, where six cases were reported by June 6. A house-to-house search of homes in the areas that were first affected uncovered a total of thirty cases that had begun in May or early June. By June 8, with six new cases and increased requests for laboratory confirmation of polio diagnoses, the Health Department realized that an epidemic might be underway. The official report on the epidemic later attributed the delay in recognizing the onset of the epidemic to physicians who delayed reporting their diagnoses of polio and to the difficulty of a correct diagnosis in the early stages of the disease. In the second week of June the Health Department increased their house inspections in affected areas and uncovered additional cases of polio. In addition, several mothers had brought their infants to a Baby Health Center in Brooklyn because their children had developed weakness and lameness in their arms or legs after having been ill for a few days. Given these additional cases, on June 17 the Health Department issued its first press notice on the rise in the number of polio cases in the city. Physicians in Brooklyn, which seemed to be the center of the epidemic, were also asked to be alert for new cases and to cooperate in controlling the disease. At the end of the month the city Health Department notified the U.S. Public Health Service, the New York State Department of Health, and the health departments of neighboring states and communities that a polio epidemic had begun (Emerson, 1917, pp. 12–15).

As word began to spread about the polio epidemic through the news media and other channels, anxiety increased among parents fearful that their children would succumb to the disease. Parents worried about their children being exposed to the disease anxiously scanned any sick child for signs of weakness or paralysis. Many also looked for a cause for the epidemic, and suspicion often fell on the many immigrants who lived in New York. Middle-class parents, in particular, were likely to blame immigrants, especially Italian immigrants, who lived in crowded, often filthy, and unsanitary conditions, for bringing the disease to the city and spreading it. Parents in the wealthier parts of the city urged the Health Department to place restrictions on immigrant communities and on the freedom of individual immigrants to move about the city as ways to limit the spread of polio. Immigrant families feared both the disease and the imminent imposition of restrictions, and repeatedly begged health officials for medical assistance for their sick infants.

Public health officials responded to the growing epidemic in several ways. On June 24, the Department of Health issued a bulletin for parents outlining what was known about polio and what they could do in the home to limit the spread of the disease. Four days later, the Board of Health passed resolutions requiring eight weeks of isolation instead of six. It also required that all patients who could not be properly quarantined at home be hospitalized. Many families could not meet the stringent quarantine requirements, which increased hospital admissions as the epidemic grew. The Health Department struggled to find sufficient hospital beds for all the patients and relied on private hospitals and the opening of new isolation hospitals to meet the increased demand. The Department also began a campaign to educate physicians about the disease so they could make accurate diagnoses and provide proper care for their patients. Hoping to slow the spread of the disease, the Health Department in early July announced several measures to prevent children from becoming infected. On July 5, the Department closed all theaters and movie houses to children under sixteen. Three days later, they prohibited all street carnivals, parades, public picnics, and excursions. Many of these restrictions remained in effect until September 29. Following a meeting of city department heads on July 9, the New York mayor issued a statement on July 10 requiring residents to clean up their garbage on a daily basis and to increase street-cleaning efforts, both in hope of reducing the spread of the disease (Emerson, 1917, pp. 15–27).

One of the more intriguing campaigns the Department of Health launched was an effort to encourage New Yorkers to "swat the fly" as part of the cleanliness crusade. Flies were thought to carry the germs that caused polio, so reducing or eliminating them would, they believed, help end the epidemic. As polio spread to children in the wealthier parts of the city, flies provided a plausible explanation of how the disease could spread out of the poorer, dirtier neighborhoods. Flies were no respecters of class and income. Families were urged to cover garbage and food so as not to attract flies, to screen their windows and doors to keep flies out, and, of course, to swat them when they could. The medical and scientific communities were divided on whether flies actually carried and transmitted polio, but it proved popular with public health officials and the general public, who felt relieved that they could do something positive to reduce the risk of polio (Rogers, 1992, pp. 57–69).

The New York Department of Health found it especially difficult to convince parents, especially immigrant parents, of the need to send their children to isolation hospitals following a diagnosis of polio. In theory, children could be quarantined at home, but no immigrant family living in a tenement could meet the stringent requirements for quarantine. These requirements included a private toilet for the family, a special room for the patient and an attendant, daily doctor visits, and separate dining facilities for the afflicted person. Families, however, feared the city hospitals given their long-standing reputation as havens for the poor and dying. They feared that if their children were hospitalized in these institutions, they would never come out alive. The New York Health Commissioner, Haven Emerson, tried to assure parents that these hospitals were clean, safe, and the best places for children with polio to receive the care they needed. Emerson also pointed out that hospitalizing the ill child reduced the chances that other children would become infected. But some parents were not convinced. Mothers sometimes hid sick children from the health authorities, and the police were occasionally called to restrain members of the family so that a sick child could be carried to the ambulance and taken to the hospital (Rogers, 1992, pp. 40–42).

As the epidemic in New York grew, and as cases began to appear in neighboring states and communities, other cities and states instituted restrictions on travelers from New York, especially on those traveling with children or suspected of fleeing the city for the presumably safer countryside. Public health authorities in these other jurisdictions wanted to prevent anyone from bringing polio into their communities. In response to these restrictions, the New York Health Department in July offered to provide certificates certifying that adults and children seeking to travel were free of polio. These certificates were provided to individuals and families after medical inspection by a physician. By the end of the epidemic, the Health Department had issued some 68,000 free-of-polio certificates and denied only 348. Not all communities, however, accepted the certificates, and even some families with certificates were barred from entry or from staying in neighboring towns and cities (Rogers, 1992, pp. 36–38).

The number of polio cases in New York City grew rapidly in June and early July. There were only 33 new cases of polio in the week ending on June 3, but this rose to 99 cases in the week ending June 17 and 445 cases for the week ending July 1. The new cases continued to rise in July, with 759 new cases for the week ending July 15 and 1,076 cases for the week ending July 29. The following week produced the largest number of new cases (1,206) for the entire epidemic. These two weeks were the peak of the epidemic. After the first week in August, the numbers began to decline, with 759 for the week ending August 19 and 367 for the week ending September 2. The number of new cases dropped below one 100 (86) for the first time since late June during the week ending October 7. Finally, the week ending November 18 saw only six cases in the city. The epidemic had burned itself out (Emerson, 1917, p. 103).

As was noted above, the 1916 epidemic occurred throughout the northeast and middle Atlantic states, although New York and New York City were the epicenters of the outbreak. Outside of the city, New York State saw 4,155 cases in 1916, of which 81 were fatal. By mid-August, New Jersey had over 1,700 cases, with over 1,300 in Newark alone. Connecticut and Pennsylvania each had over 300 cases, and significant numbers of cases were reported in Ohio, Rhode Island, Kansas, Illinois, Wisconsin, and Massachusetts (Rogers, 1992, pp. 11, 191 n. 5).

All told, the 1916 epidemic was one of the most severe in the history of polio in the United States. The polio rate that year was 41.1 per 100,000 population, the worst in American history. However, the total number of cases, 27,000, was substantially fewer than the 57,000 in 1952. Because the population of the United States had increased substantially since 1916, the polio rate in 1952 was only 37.2 per 100,000 (Historical Statistics, 1975, p. 77; "Incidence Rates," 1999, p. 3). A disease that had barely registered on the public consciousness before 1900, polio had suddenly become a major worry for parents, physicians, and public health officials alike.

Part of what made the 1916 epidemic so frightening, apart from the sheer number of patients, was that so little was known about a disease that could quickly paralyze a healthy youngster or adult. Although the virus that causes polio had been discovered a few years earlier, doctors still had no clear idea how it was transmitted from patients to new victims, why it paralyzed some victims and left others virtually untouched, or how to prevent new infections. Doctors also had no way to intervene once a child was infected; the disease simply had to run its course while doctors made the patient comfortable and hoped that any paralysis would be minimal. If parents often felt helpless when their child was stricken, many physicians felt no less so. All anyone could do was wait, hope, and pray. Still, scientists and physicians had begun to unlock polio's secrets, even though what they had learned by 1916 was no help in ending the epidemic.

3

Science, Medicine, and the Search for a Cure

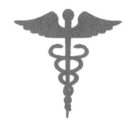

T he growing prevalence of polio in the early twentieth century caught the attention of scientific and medical researchers in both Europe and the United States. Beginning in the 1890s sanitation improved in northern Europe and the United States, and polio began making the shift from an endemic disease to an epidemic one. Small epidemics occurred with increasing frequency, and the number of cases in these epidemics began to climb. At the outset of scientific research into the disease, little was known other than it seemed to be contagious and obviously capable of causing permanent paralysis. No one knew what caused the disease, how it spread from person to person, why some people recovered with little permanent damage and others were paralyzed for life or died, or why infants and children were most likely to come down with polio. Although some of these questions would be answered by scientific research in the early decades of the twentieth century, polio only slowly gave up its secrets to medical investigators.

IVAR WICKMAN AND SWEDISH RESEARCH

Some of the earliest scientific research into this newly emergent disease was conducted by scientists in Sweden, which had experienced polio epidemics in

1899, in 1903, and in 1905, when there were 1,031 cases in the largest world epidemic up to that time. Ivar Wickman, a young Swedish doctor and epidemiologist, observed the 1899 and 1903 epidemics as a medical assistant in a Stockholm clinic. When the 1905 epidemic erupted, Wickman decided to study the outbreak to see what he could discover about polio, the way it spread, and how contagious it was. As he began his study, Wickman made a crucial decision to include abortive, non-paralytic, and paralytic polio cases in his study. This decision would enable him to get a more accurate picture of the extent of the disease and how it spread in a community (Paul, 1971, pp. 88–89).

Wickman's study of the 1905 epidemic revealed a number of interesting characteristics of polio. Relatively isolated rural communities in Sweden experienced much higher rates of polio than the more crowded cities. Wickman believed this was because children in these communities had no previous exposure to the disease and thus no immunity when polio struck. His study also revealed that polio was not just a disease of the central nervous system; mild cases in which there was no paralysis, and hence no nervous system involvement, also helped spread the disease. Wickman also estimated that the incubation period for the disease, the time between infection and the beginning of disease symptoms, was three to four days, a figure that would only be confirmed in the 1950s. Wickman's most important conclusion was that polio was a very contagious disease in which mild, non-paralytic cases were just as important as the paralytic ones in spreading the illness (Paul, 1971, pp. 89–95).

Unfortunately, Wickman's study did not have the immediate impact it deserved. The discovery of the poliovirus a few years later encouraged scientists to focus their studies on experimental polio rather than on the knowledge that could be gained from careful epidemiological and clinical studies. Scientists studying experimental polio concentrated on the actions of the virus in nerve tissue, especially in the spinal cord, which, while important information, did not address some important facts about how polio entered humans, where it went, and what it did before it damaged the nerves of the spinal cord. It would not be until the 1930s that scientists again took a careful look at what epidemiological and clinical research could reveal about how the poliovirus entered the body and what it did once it gained entry.

KARL LANDSTEINER AND THE DISCOVERY OF THE POLIOVIRUS

The next important step in understanding polio came in the laboratory of the Vienna, Austria, immunologist Dr. Karl Landsteiner. Landsteiner, along with his assistant Erwin Popper, would be the first to identify the cause of polio as what was then called a filterable virus. Virology, the study of viruses, was in its infancy in the early twentieth century. Only a few viruses, including those causing smallpox and rabies, had been identified when Landsteiner discovered the poliovirus in 1908. Part of the problem was that viruses were too small to be seen by even the most powerful optical microscopes of the time. The only way to identify a virus was to pass suspected infected material taken from someone with the disease through filters with holes too small to permit the passage of all known bacteria. If the material that had passed through the filters was then injected into a laboratory animal such as a monkey and appeared to cause the same disease as that in the individual or animal from which the material was taken, the scientist could conclude that the disease was caused by a filterable virus too small to be seen.

In 1908 Landsteiner and Popper ground up spinal cord material from the body of a nine-year-old boy who had died of polio and suspended it in a sterile fluid. This fluid was then injected into rabbits, guinea pigs, and mice. There was no change in the health of these experimental animals because these animals are not susceptible to the human poliovirus. However, the two scientists also injected the material into the abdomens of two different types of monkeys, who, fortunately for medical science, were susceptible to the virus. The first monkey developed an illness after six days and died on the eighth day following the injection without showing any obvious signs of paralysis. The second monkey's legs were completely paralyzed following an illness seventeen days after receiving the shot. When the monkeys were autopsied, cross-sections of their spinal cords showed the same kind of damage found in cross-sections of the spinal cord of the young boy who had died and from whom the injected material had come. Although this was not a definitive experiment, the two researchers had provided pretty good evidence that polio was caused by a virus that could be isolated from the nervous tissue of individuals with the disease. They announced their discovery at a medical meeting in Vienna and published their results soon after (Paul, 1971, pp. 98–100).

Once Landsteiner's and Popper's results were published, other experimenters in Europe and the United States repeated the experiment and confirmed their results. Their discovery encouraged other scientists to concentrate on studying polio in the laboratory to better understand how it entered the body and did its damage to the spinal cord. In experiments conducted over the next several years, researchers in several countries were able to detect poliovirus in non-nervous tissues collected from humans who had died of the disease. They found evidence of the poliovirus in tissues taken from tonsils, from the lining of the throat, in nasal secretions, in salivary glands, and in intestinal lymph nodes. This evidence supported Wickman's belief derived from his epidemiological studies that polio was more than just a disease of the central nervous system, even if that was where the damage that caused paralysis was done. Researchers, including Landsteiner and Popper, were also soon able to take material from the spinal cord of a monkey infected with human polio virus, prepare a solution, and inject it into yet other monkeys. That these new monkeys developed polio as a result of passing the virus from monkey to monkey was additional evidence confirming the original identification of the poliovirus (Paul, 1971, pp. 100–102).

THE POLIO RESEARCH OF DR. SIMON FLEXNER

When news of Landsteiner's and Popper's discovery of the poliovirus reached New York, Dr. Simon Flexner, director of the Rockefeller Institute for Medical Research, was eager to use the resources of his facility to study the microorganism. Flexner's interest in polio had increased due to his participation on the committee that studied the 1907 polio epidemic in New York. The Rockefeller Institute was well funded and well equipped to work with viruses. They also had the money to be able to house and work with monkeys, which were much more expensive and required more care than other laboratory animals. Since many traditional laboratory animals were not susceptible to polio, Flexner needed to work with primates if he was going to make progress in his study of the poliovirus.

Shortly after receiving news of the discovery in Vienna, Flexner and his colleagues were able to replicate the work of the Austrian scientists. They took spinal cord material from two fatal cases of polio in New Jersey and New York, prepared and filtered the material, and injected it into monkeys. Their results were similar to those obtained earlier by Landsteiner and Popper and mark the first isolation of poliovirus in the United States. Flexner and Dr. Martha Wollstein also succeeded in passing the two strains of poliovirus from monkey to monkey, thus providing further proof when the animals were autopsied that the virus caused the damage observed. Flexner's early success convinced him that the way in which the poliovirus operated in the laboratory monkeys was the way it operated in humans (Paul, 1971, pp. 107–108). Unfortunately, Flexner's assumptions eventually proved wrong, and his early laboratory successes and the prestige of his position sent polio research down the wrong track for several decades.

Flexner and his team at the Rockefeller Institute followed their isolation of the poliovirus with numerous experiments that they hoped would reveal how polio was spread, how it entered the body, and how it entered and damaged the central nervous system. Scientists at the Rockefeller Institute and in laboratories in Europe also tried to identify where in the body the virus could be found outside the spinal cord. Knowing this would be important to devising any plan of immunization. Flexner and his colleagues succeeded in demonstrating that serum derived from the blood of monkeys recovering from experimental poliomyelitis contained antibodies to the poliovirus. Shortly after Flexner's discovery of antibodies in monkeys, French scientists demonstrated that humans recovering from polio also produced antibodies to the poliovirus (Paul, 1971, pp. 115–116). These discoveries were important because they demonstrated that the immune system could be stimulated to produce antibodies against the virus through a vaccine. The antibodies, whether acquired in response to a natural infection or immunization, would protect the individual from developing the disease if he or she was exposed to the poliovirus in the future.

By 1913 it was clear to Flexner and his colleagues that it would be very difficult to protect humans against polio or to cure the disease. While doctors had learned a great deal following Landsteiner's discovery of the poliovirus, much remained to be learned about the behavior of the virus within the body and about the ways in which it was spread. However, Flexner's emphasis on studying polio experimentally in the laboratory put impediments in the way of uncovering polio's secrets. Flexner was firmly committed to his belief that polio was solely a disease of the central nervous system. He came to this conviction because of his success in producing polio in monkeys by injecting the virus into the nerves in the noses of the animals. From there the virus traveled to the spinal cord, where it damaged and destroyed the anterior horn cells that were crucial to the working of the neurons that controlled muscle movement. Flexner believed polio entered humans through the nose and then into the nervous system, although for ethical reasons he could not test his theory directly on humans because of the potentially devastating consequences of a case of polio. It would take a different kind of evidence from epidemiological and clinical studies to reveal that the mouth, not the nose, was the usual entry point for the virus, and that research would not be undertaken until the 1930s.

CLINICAL STUDIES IN SWEDEN

In 1911 Sweden experienced another serious polio epidemic with 3,840 cases, far exceeding any previous polio epidemics in the world. Swedish scientists took advantage of the unfortunate opportunity provided by the epidemic to conduct additional clinical and epidemiological research. A group of scientists at a bacteriological institute in Stockholm carried out a number of tests on patients with polio. In autopsies of patients who had died of the disease, the Swedish doctors isolated the poliovirus from several different sites within the bodies. Again, this indicated that the poliovirus existed outside of nerve tissue. Even more importantly, for the first time they succeeded in isolating poliovirus from living patients. They found the virus from patients in both the acute and convalescent stages of the disease as well as in children with mild and inapparent infections. This was important because it confirmed Ivar Wickman's theory that polio could be spread just as easily by those with mild or inapparent infections as by those with severe paralytic polio. Although the Swedish researchers published their findings and presented their results at medical conferences, for a variety of reasons their results were largely ignored while other scientists such as Flexner pursued the study of polio in the laboratory. It was only in the 1930s that this early work on polio would be rediscovered and largely confirmed by new studies (Paul, 1971, pp. 126–131).

By the time of the major New York epidemic of 1916, doctors and scientists knew a fair amount about the organism that caused polio. They knew it was caused by a filterable virus and that it had a predilection for nerve tissue, which was where it did the damage that caused the characteristic paralysis. If they read the medical literature carefully, especially that coming out of Sweden, they knew that even individuals with very mild or inapparent polio were contagious and could transmit the disease. And while Flexner and others supported the nose as the portal of entry, the fact that the poliovirus could be isolated from tissues taken from the throat and intestine suggested that the mouth, not the nose, might be the way the virus entered the body. But doctors were still a long way from fully understanding the poliovirus and how it caused paralysis and death. And nothing they had discovered by 1916, as we have seen, helped prevent the great epidemic that year or cure those who came down with polio.

4

Franklin D. Roosevelt, Polio, and Warm Springs

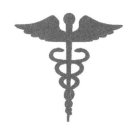

Following its emergence as an epidemic disease in the late nineteenth century, polio was most often known as "infantile paralysis," for the vast majority of its victims were infants and young children. Doctors had treated adolescents and even adults for infantile paralysis, but these cases were unusual. This popular and medical idea of infantile paralysis as a disease of young children received a jolt in 1921 when a rising Democratic politician named Franklin D. Roosevelt contracted polio at the age of thirty-nine. Roosevelt (aka FDR) seemed to have a bright future ahead of him. The only child of a wealthy New York couple, he was a graduate of Harvard University and Columbia University Law School and had married a distant cousin, Eleanor Roosevelt. FDR had been elected to the New York State Senate in 1910 and would serve there until appointed Assistant Secretary of the Navy by President Woodrow Wilson in March 1913. Roosevelt resigned in August 1920 to run for Vice President of the United States on the Democratic ticket with James M. Cox. Cox and Roosevelt were badly beaten by the Republicans Warren G. Harding and Calvin Coolidge, but Roosevelt had campaigned hard, made many contacts and friends, and emerged from the election as a young Democratic politician with lots of promise. Following his defeat, Roosevelt took a job in New York with the Fidelity & Deposit Company, a firm that guaranteed private and government contracts. Roosevelt made five times what he had made in government service, and the position allowed him to maintain his law practice and to give political speeches. Roosevelt seemed well positioned to make another bid for national office, but in July 1921 he began a trip north to the family vacation home on Campobello Island off the coast of Maine that would alter his life forever.

ROOSEVELT AND POLIO

In late July 1921, Franklin Roosevelt and about fifty other men traveled north from New York City to inspect a Boy Scout Camp at Bear Mountain on the Hudson River. It was the kind of event the outgoing Roosevelt relished, with its parades, speeches, and participation in scout activities. Most Roosevelt biographers believe that it was during his visit to the scout encampment that FDR was infected with the poliovirus. Because he had led a very sheltered childhood, it was likely that he had never been exposed to polio as a young child, and thus it had devastating consequences when he encountered it as an adult.

On August 5, Roosevelt set sail for Campobello Island on the yacht *Sabalo* with the yacht's owner, Van-Lear Black, his boss at Fidelity and Deposit. Two days later they arrived at the island. On August 10 Roosevelt took his wife and two sons sailing in the bay. The family saw smoke rising off one of the small islands and landed to put the fire out. The family was covered with soot and dirt while fighting the fire and when they returned to their cottage, Roosevelt was feeling somewhat weak, but he set off across the island with his children to swim in a freshwater pond two miles away. After swimming in the warm water of the pond, the family dove into the cold water of the Bay of Fundy. Roosevelt then raced his two boys back to the cottage. He was so tired when he got home that he didn't even take off his wet swimming suit when he sat down to read the mail.

He began to feel feverish and his wife urged him to go to bed to rest. He ate little of the food sent up to him and was restless all night. In the morning, he nearly fell going to the bathroom, but he shaved and managed to get back to bed. He seemed to be getting sicker instead of better, and when Eleanor took his temperature, it was 102°F. The pain in his back increased, and paralysis began to affect both legs. Eleanor called in a local physician, who thought Roosevelt had a bad cold, a diagnosis FDR knew was wrong. The next morning, Friday, Roosevelt could not stand without assistance, and Eleanor and Louis Howe, Roosevelt's aide, searched for another doctor who could give a second, and perhaps more informed, opinion. They found Dr. William Keen in Bar Harbor, but he was unable to reach Campobello until Sunday morning.

He diagnosed Roosevelt's illness as a blood clot on the spinal cord that was causing his inability to move his legs. The doctor expected Roosevelt to recover and instructed Eleanor and Louis Howe to massage FDR's legs. The massages, which the two administered over the next two days, were extremely painful and did nothing to impede the progress of the paralysis, which soon affected everything below Roosevelt's waist including his bowels and his bladder. By Monday Roosevelt was delirious with a still rising fever. Then the fever broke, although the pain remained.

As Roosevelt's agony continued, Louis Howe and Eleanor consulted with family members in New York, who in turn described FDR's symptoms to specialists. These specialists suspected that Roosevelt might have infantile paralysis. The family then arranged for Dr. Robert W. Lovett, a Boston physician and an authority on polio, to come to Campobello to examine Roosevelt. Lovett finally arrived at the cottage on August 25, two weeks after the onset of paralysis in Roosevelt's legs. Lovett examined Roosevelt carefully since his patient's muscles were still very painful. He noted that Roosevelt's arms were weak, that his face seemed partially paralyzed, and that his legs were extremely weak, especially near the hips. Following his examination, Lovett informed the family that Roosevelt indeed had polio. In Lovett's opinion, it was a mild case, but only time would tell. The painful massage was to be stopped immediately, as it might further damage the affected muscles. The only thing Roosevelt and the others could do was wait to see how much permanent damage the disease would do. Roosevelt grew discouraged after Lovett departed because his leg muscles continued to weaken and because there was nothing that could be done to stem the spread of paralysis.

Because Roosevelt was already a public figure, Louis Howe and Eleanor Roosevelt knew that word would soon get out about FDR's illness, and they tried to manage the news so as to minimize the public's knowledge about the seriousness of his sickness and the extent of paralysis. The first newspaper notice that appeared on August 27 did not mention infantile paralysis and stressed FDR's quick recovery. Back on Campobello, Roosevelt's muscle weakness continued, and he resisted Dr. Lovett's instructions not to try to move or exercise his legs even though exercise at this early stage of recovery would make the permanent damage worse. With the fever gone and Roosevelt feeling somewhat better, he, Eleanor and Louis Howe made plans to return him to New York. On September 13, Roosevelt was lifted onto a stretcher and carried by six men down the stairs of his cottage, across the porch, and down the sloping lawn to the dock, where he was placed in a small boat to take him across the bay to Maine. Roosevelt's muscles were still extremely tender and every jostle and wave were very painful, but he did not complain. FDR's traveling companions had to take a window out of the private train car in which he would travel to get the stretcher into the train. Finally, Roosevelt was placed in his berth. Louis Howe had distracted curious reporters by directing them to another dock in Maine, and the media arrived at the train only after Roosevelt was on board. As the train pulled out of the station, the reporters and villagers saw Roosevelt through the window of the train smiling and smoking a cigarette.

ROOSEVELT'S REHABILITATION

Roosevelt returned to New York on September 14 and was taken by ambulance to New York Presbyterian Hospital. There he came under the care of Dr. Lovett's protégé, Dr. George Draper, who would himself become a leading expert on the care and rehabilitation of poliomyelitis patients. On September 16 the *New York Times* published a front-page article that for the first time publicly disclosed that Roosevelt was ill with infantile paralysis. The article minimized the extent of his paralysis and held out hope for his full recovery.

Roosevelt's spirits were good on his return to New York, but he was so weak that all but immediate family members were barred from his hospital room. He still occasionally had a fever, his muscles remained very tender, and the paralysis remained. Some of the affected muscles began to show signs of atrophy. Dr. Draper was concerned about Roosevelt's slow recovery and the failure of many of the muscles to show any improvement, especially in his back and legs. Roosevelt did regain the ability to use his hands, although his shoulders and arms remained weak. But the legs failed to respond to FDR's efforts to move them. Draper was also concerned that Roosevelt's overly optimistic belief that he would make a complete and quick recovery could lead to depression once Roosevelt grasped the severity of the situation and realized that he very likely would not regain the use of his legs. As Roosevelt's strength and mood began slowly to improve, his children and selected friends were able to visit him in the hospital. Roosevelt always met them with a smile and was upbeat about the prospects for his complete recovery, even as his doctors remained concerned about the extent of permanent paralysis. Soon FDR was able to sit up, as his back muscles were less seriously impaired than the doctors had feared. His leg muscles, however, showed no signs of recovery. Nonetheless, Drs. Draper and Lovett decided Roosevelt had recovered sufficiently to return to his New York house, which he did on October 28. He was carried up the stairs and installed in the quietest bedroom in the house.

Dr. Lovett arranged for Roosevelt to begin physical therapy to try to regain the use of the affected muscles. On December 1, 1921, he began working with Kathleen Lake. Unlike many polio patients who resisted the hard work of rehabilitation, FDR was eager to begin. Even the often painful exercises were better than lying immobile all day. Lake stretched Roosevelt's stiff muscles every day except Sunday. Roosevelt endured the painful stretching of his contracted muscles with his usual good cheer. He was also willing to go slowly, as prescribed by Lovett, rather than charging ahead in his usual fashion.

With the New Year, Roosevelt began spending time in his room working on both Democratic Party correspondence and his work with Fidelity & Deposit. His exercises continued under the supervision of Kathleen Lake. In late January, Roosevelt experienced a setback when the hamstring muscles of his legs tightened, pulling his knees toward his chest. Draper and a colleague decided to encase FDR's bent legs in plaster, with an opening cut behind the knees. Each day wedges were forced into the opening, slowly forcing Roosevelt's legs to straighten. Roosevelt experienced unrelieved pain for two weeks during this procedure. When the casts came off in mid-February, Roosevelt's muscles had largely atrophied. He had virtually no strength in either of his lower legs. It was clear that he would not be able to stand unassisted, and he was measured for steel braces. Roosevelt's leather and steel braces weighed fourteen pounds and stretched from his heel to his waist, including a leather pelvic band around his waist.

Seven months after he was stricken with polio, surrounded by Mrs. Lake, Dr. Draper, his nurse, and the family butler, Roosevelt stood for the first time in his braces. They slid crutches under his arms to help him balance and move about the room. Because his legs and hips were paralyzed, FDR had to learn to walk using the muscles of his upper body. Though in constant danger of falling, being upright and able to move, even slowly and awkwardly, raised Roosevelt's spirits. While strength was returning to some of Roosevelt's muscles in his upper legs, his lower legs showed no signs of recovery.

In May, Roosevelt, along with his nurse and valet, moved from New York City to his mother's home, Springwood, in Hyde Park, north along the Hudson River. His wife and children followed once the school term ended. At Hyde Park, Roosevelt continued his rehabilitation under the direction of Kathleen Lake, who now came three days a week. Sara Roosevelt hoped that her son would stay permanently at Springwood, where he could recover from his illness. When Eleanor and the children joined FDR in June, the tension in the Roosevelt household increased. Eleanor encouraged her husband to push on with his exercises so as to hasten his recovery. His mother encouraged him to rest and to resist the urge to resume a more active life. Eleanor and Sara Roosevelt had had from the very beginning a difficult relationship, and now that relationship threatened to interfere with FDR's recovery. Drs. Draper and Lovett decided that the only remedy was to remove Roosevelt from his family for a while and in late June arranged for him to go to Boston where Lovett could examine him and have him fitted for new braces.

Dr. Lovett's examination of Roosevelt in Boston revealed that his back muscles were recovering nicely, but there was little recovery in his leg muscles. While Lovett could do little to restore Roosevelt's paralyzed muscles, he did arrange for one of his assistants, Wilhemine Wright, to teach Roosevelt how to use crutches more effectively. Wright instructed FDR on how to rise out of a chair while in his braces and how to negotiate a set of stairs. Roosevelt learned to do both, but rising out of a chair alone was awkward and embarrassing in public and using stairs was both difficult and dangerous, especially if there were no railings. Once he returned to public life, FDR tried to minimize these activities so as not to draw attention to his disability.

Once he returned to Hyde Park in July, Roosevelt continued to work hard to recover the use of his legs. He worked with Kathleen Lake three mornings a week, and she encouraged him to swim in warm water. Roosevelt discovered that, aided by the buoyancy of the water, he could move more easily. When the water of the pool at Springwood proved too cold for Roosevelt, his friend Vincent Astor offered him the use of his heated pool. Roosevelt had parallel bars erected on the lawn at his home so that he could try to build strength in his legs by walking back and forth between them. Dr. Lovett also urged him to continue to practice his walking with his braces and crutches. Even though his upper-body strength had largely returned, crutch walking was difficult for Roosevelt. He walked down the quarter mile drive of Springwood toward the main road, but the effort exhausted him. He apparently made it to the end of the drive only once.

By 1923 Roosevelt began to settle into a routine that he followed until his return to active political life in 1928. He retained his position with Fidelity & Deposit, although he was often absent from the office. Roosevelt left his law firm and established a new law practice with Basil O'Connor, a relationship that would have profound impact on the history of polio in America. But much of his time was spent trying to regain the use of his legs. For a while he continued his exercises under the supervision of Drs. Lovett and Draper, but Roosevelt was also open to all sorts of unorthodox and unproven suggestions. He also purchased a used houseboat in Florida, which he named the *Larooco*, and he spent several winters on the boat with friends. Roosevelt had discovered that the warm Florida sun and the warm waters of the state were good for his muscles and his mood. However, as much as good sailing and swimming in the warm waters did for Roosevelt's disposition, they did not bring his legs back to life.

In the summer of 1924 Roosevelt received a letter from George Foster Peabody, a financier who had contributed to FDR's political campaigns.

Peabody had purchased an interest in the Meriwether Inn in Warm Springs, Georgia. The inn was a decrepit resort set among the warm mineral springs some seventy miles southwest of Atlanta. Included with Peabody's letter was Louis Joseph's account of how the warm mineral waters at the resort had brought his polio-paralyzed legs back to life. After three summers of swimming in and walking across the bottom of the pools, Joseph was able to leave his wheelchair and walk with only two canes. Roosevelt decided to visit Warm Springs on his trip south in October.

ROOSEVELT AND WARM SPRINGS

Roosevelt arrived in Warm Springs by train in early October 1924. Although the condition of the resort was depressing, Roosevelt was eager to try the pools. On his first morning in Warm Springs, Louis Joseph walked into Roosevelt's room using only one cane. He described for FDR how he had strengthened his leg muscles by walking in the warm pools. Roosevelt was impressed and with the aid of his valet took his first plunge into the pool that very afternoon. He moved about the pool and was impressed by how the buoyant water made every movement easier. During his first two-week stay in Warm Springs, Roosevelt thought about buying the resort, restoring its faded grandeur, and providing a place for polio survivors to benefit from the healing mineral water. Others, including Basil O'Connor and Eleanor Roosevelt, worried about the cost of the venture, but Roosevelt himself remained upbeat about the possibilities.

Toward the end of Roosevelt's first visit to Warm Springs a reporter from the *Atlanta Journal* wrote an article for the paper's Sunday supplement. The lead article described Roosevelt's efforts to swim his way back to a full recovery. Roosevelt praised the warm water for making it easier for him to move while in the pool, and he claimed to be benefiting substantially from both the warm water and the warm Georgia sun. The article also noted that Roosevelt intended to return in the spring of 1925 to stay for several months. The article was widely reprinted in newspapers across the country and started many polio survivors thinking about how they, too, could get to Warm Springs and recover alongside Roosevelt.

In early February 1925, Roosevelt traveled south once again to spend several weeks aboard his houseboat in Florida. Then in early April he returned to Warm Springs. To his surprise, he learned that numerous polio survivors had contacted Tom Loyless, who was managing the resort. Most wanted to learn how they could benefit from the healing springs. Others were bolder and simply arrived by train in Warm Springs. Loyless turned some of these early arrivals away since there were no facilities or staff to assist them. Roosevelt initially resented the intrusion of these other polio survivors on his recovery, but soon decided that he had an obligation to see what could be done to help them since it was his enthusiastic recommendation of the springs that had brought them to Georgia.

Roosevelt had no training in physiotherapy beyond his own experience with physical therapy. And in his case, four years of exercise in water and on land had brought little improvement in his paralyzed legs. Nonetheless, Roosevelt resolved to see what he could do for the small number of polio survivors who had come to be healed. He asked a physician from a neighboring town to examine each of the visitors. Roosevelt then tested the muscles of each polio survivor using the method Dr. Lovett had used on him. Once in the pool, Roosevelt devised simple exercises for each of the survivors to perform in the warm spring water. He had a railing installed in the pool for the swimmers to hold on to, and an underwater platform for exercise. Roosevelt also hired two local boys to help the men and women in and out of the pool. With his infectious smile and gracious manner, Roosevelt also addressed the emotional devastation most polio survivors experienced. He was determined that the mood at Warm Springs would always be more like that of a resort than the grim state institutions where most polio survivors had been rehabilitated. He demonstrated that recovery from polio could be full of smiles and laughter as well as pain and hard work.

The regular customers began to return to Warm Springs when the resort season opened on May 1. However, they were unhappy to see the resort seemingly taken over by men and women clanking down the halls in braces and on crutches or wheeling themselves around the grounds in the large wicker wheelchairs. Needing to keep the resort visitors to help pay the bills, Roosevelt and Loyless arranged to have a second dining room opened for the polio survivors, hastened the repair of the cottages so that the main inn building would be reserved for resort patrons, and began a second and smaller pool for the therapeutic exercises. These efforts didn't please all the guests of the resort and many left. Their departure confirmed in Roosevelt his intention to transform the resort into a first-class polio rehabilitation facility.

In the spring of 1926, Roosevelt took a final cruise on his houseboat in Florida before turning his full attention to matters at Warm Springs. Tom Loyless had died of cancer, so FDR was now in charge of everything. There were twenty-three polio survivors expecting to be healed, the facilities still needed substantial repair, and it wasn't at all clear whether a polio rehabilitation facility operated like a resort could be made to work financially. Roosevelt also convinced Dr. Leroy W. Hubbard, head of rehabilitation for the New York

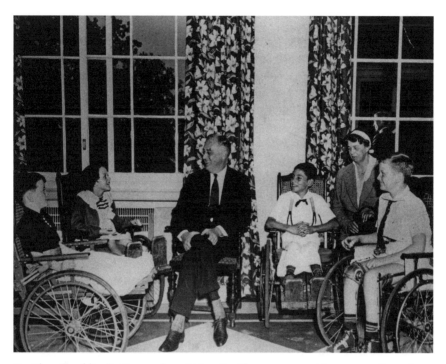

President Franklin D. Roosevelt and his wife, Eleanor, meet with young polio patients undergoing rehabilitation at the Georgia Warm Springs Foundation in 1933. (March of Dimes)

State Department of Public Health, to come to Warm Springs to direct the rehabilitation program. Hubbard brought with him Helena T. Mahoney, a physiotherapist who would become a fixture at Warm Springs. Roosevelt also decided to buy Warm Springs at a cost of $195,000, nearly two thirds of his wealth. Both Eleanor and Basil O'Connor opposed the risky purchase, but FDR was determined, and after complicated negotiations with George Peabody the deal was finalized. Roosevelt now owned a failing resort that he hoped to turn into a facility where polio survivors could rehabilitate both their bodies and their spirits.

When he returned to Warm Springs in September 1926, Roosevelt was both the owner and chief inspiration for a new kind of rehabilitation facility. He would spend about half his time over the next two years transforming the place. He had a new cottage built for himself and began to address the many challenges facing him. He put the rehabilitation program in the hands of Dr. Hubbard and Helena Mahoney and concentrated on renovating the old resort and finding the money to pay for it. He had hoped to build a first-class resort and rehabilitation facility, but resort guests didn't want to vacation with a group of polio survivors undergoing rehabilitation, so he soon eliminated the non-polio part of the resort. His goal of creating a rehabilitation facility received a boost in January 1927, when the American Orthopedic Association assessed the work of Hubbard and Mahoney and recommended the establishment of a polio rehabilitation center at Warm Springs.

With the aid of his law partner, Basil O'Connor, Roosevelt established the Georgia Warm Springs Foundation to raise money to support the new facility. He oversaw all the details of transforming the resort into an accessible and welcoming place. Eighty new patients arrived in 1927, which posed a challenge for the staff of the unfinished establishment. Roosevelt also established the rules for Warm Springs. He wanted no uniformed attendants because that would make it too much like a hospital, and he wanted to maintain the atmosphere of a resort. FDR imbued the place with his optimistic, out going approach to life and recovery. One physiotherapist recalled "There *were* no back bedrooms for polios at Warm Springs.... He meant it to be *their* world, no one else's." A patient recalled that Warm Springs was "just a wonderful place to be," and he gave all the credit to Roosevelt: "He was the kind of man who would come into a room and make it his. When he came in, the *dynamo* was there." Another patient remembered that FDR's "greatest contribution was himself ... the apparent ease with which he handled himself" (Ward, 1989, p. 771). Hugh Gallagher, a polio patient, had not wanted to go to Warm Springs, but he discovered once there that it "was the best thing ever to happen" to him. "The difference between life as a patient in the old hospital and rehabilitation at the beautiful resort, deep in the Georgia pines, was as great as the difference between Kansas and Oz" (Gallagher, 1998, p. 71).

The greater funding provided by the Georgia Warm Springs Foundation and the hiring of a professional staff under the direction of Dr. Hubbard turned Roosevelt's purchase into a leading polio rehabilitation facility. Polio patients from all across the country hoped to be able to travel to Georgia for their recovery, but Warm Springs served only a small portion of each epidemic's survivors. At its height, it had room for only about 100 patients at a time. Because it was in the rural south during the time of racial segregation, Warm Springs during the Roosevelt era never admitted African Americans as patients, although a number worked there in various capacities. Still, for those patients treated there, Warm Springs restored both their bodies and their spirits in the wake of polio's devastation. In addition, it served as a model for what other sites of rehabilitation could and should be.

5

Scientific Research and the First Human Vaccine Trials

Although some scientific and medical research on poliomyelitis continued during the 1920s, it was not until the 1930s that physicians and scientists began to make real progress in understanding the disease. During that decade researchers provided additional and persuasive evidence that polio was an intestinal disease and that the mouth, not the nose, was the point of entry for the virus. Scientists in Australia also provided the first convincing evidence that there were at least two different strains of polio. These successful scientific advances were diminished by the failure of the first human trials of polio vaccines in 1935. While much had been learned about polio since the discovery of the poliovirus, the disastrous 1935 vaccine trials demonstrated that medicine did not yet know enough about the virus and the disease to be able to develop a human vaccine that was both safe and effective.

REVIVAL OF CLINICAL VIROLOGY

As we saw earlier, Dr. Simon Flexner's success in isolating the poliovirus and in inducing polio experimentally in monkeys by injecting the virus into the nerves of their noses focused the research of polio on laboratory experiments.

The dominance of Flexner's approach lasted for about two decades. In the 1930s several research groups began to focus their study on how polio worked in humans. To some extent, these American scientists were continuing and expanding on the kinds of clinical studies of polio that Ivar Wickman had pioneered in Sweden early in the twentieth century. These new studies confirmed the importance of the minor forms of the illness in spreading polio in an epidemic. In addition, they provided new and convincing evidence that the mouth, not the nose, was the portal of entry for the poliovirus in humans and that, for most humans infected with the virus, polio was a relatively minor intestinal disease.

In the summer of 1931 a severe polio epidemic broke out in Connecticut and the rest of the northeastern United States. Although not as severe as the great 1916 epidemic, it nonetheless caught the attention of physicians at the Yale University School of Medicine. Dr. James D. Trask was appointed head of the newly created Yale Poliomyelitis Commission. One of the other original members was Dr. John R. Paul, who would later write a fine history of the conquest of polio. The Yale physicians decided to try to determine the role that abortive polio, a very minor illness with no paralysis, played in polio epidemics. They wanted to try to recover the poliovirus from patients who had abortive polio. They looked for a family in which there was an obvious case of polio with paralysis and in which other members of the family had experienced minor illnesses at the same time. Over the course of the summer, the Yale physicians took throat samples from twelve children suspected of having abortive polio. Two of the samples produced polio when injected into monkeys. The scientists had demonstrated that their procedure worked, but they would need much more evidence to convince themselves and a skeptical medical establishment that the mouth and throat, not the nose, were the way the poliovirus entered the body. This also marked a return to studying how polio worked in humans rather than focusing so exclusively on experimental studies with monkeys (Paul, 1971, pp. 204–207).

THE NOSE OR THE MOUTH

The question of how the poliovirus entered the body was an important one for doctors to answer with some certainty. If the nose was the entry point, it was likely that the virus circulated in the air and that someone could catch the poliovirus in ways similar to the influenza virus. If the mouth was the entry point, it was likely that the virus was swallowed and found its way into the mouth on the dirty fingers of children. Determining definitively how the poliovirus entered the body had important implications for public health measures devised to stop the spread of polio and for strategies in developing effective and safe vaccines (Paul, 1971, p. 247). In the 1930s, a number of laboratory experiments cast increasing doubt on the theory that the poliovirus entered humans through the nose. At the same time, there was growing evidence from clinical studies of polio during the epidemics of the 1930s that implicated the mouth as the portal of entry. Still, some physicians were reluctant to abandon the old orthodoxy that the nose was the portal of entry, and it was not until the mid-1940s that most physicians accepted the mouth as the most important avenue for the poliovirus to enter humans (Paul, 1971, p. 251).

Although Swedish researchers had isolated the poliovirus from fecal material of humans infected with the disease early in the century, this discovery had not been substantiated by subsequent research. However, in the 1930s new evidence emerged to support the Swedish discoveries. In 1937, a researcher in Chicago isolated the poliovirus from five of seventeen intestinal washings of polio patients. This report sparked the interest of the Yale Poliomyelitis Unit, and they decided to try to replicate the Chicago results. During a small polio epidemic in Connecticut that year, the Yale physicians took stool samples from twenty-two patients. Three of nine throat samples were positive, as were three of thirteen stool samples. In the case of one young boy who had a minor illness but whose brother had paralytic polio, the doctors were able to isolate the poliovirus from the boy's stool twenty-four days after his sickness. The scientists discovered that it was easier to detect the poliovirus in stool samples than in throat washings. There were two reasons for this: first, the virus apparently remained in the throat only briefly, and, second, there was a larger amount of the virus in the stool, and it remained in stool samples for several weeks following the acute illness. Other researchers soon confirmed the Yale results by also finding the poliovirus in stool samples. During several epidemics in 1939 and 1940, the Yale physicians isolated the poliovirus in the sewage of cities undergoing polio epidemics. Many older physicians who had long studied polio and who were loyal to the older theory that polio entered via the nose challenged the Yale findings. However, evidence continued to mount that polio was spread by fecal material and sewage contaminated by the poliovirus and that young children were the likely reservoir of the virus. It was also increasingly evident that children and adults who appeared healthy but who had been infected could also shed the virus in their stools. These discoveries would, over the next decade, alter public health measures to try to stem epidemics and foster the development of a polio vaccine (Paul, 1971, pp. 279–286).

HOW MANY STRAINS OF POLIO?

In addition to the question of how the poliovirus entered the body, scientists in the 1930s also began to explore the problem of how many strains or types of polio existed. In 1931, two Australian researchers, Frank M. Burnet and Jean McNamara, established that there were at least two genetically distinct strains of poliovirus that produced distinct antibody reactions. In a variety of experiments conducted during the 1930s, the Yale scientists used samples from American patients and confirmed the discovery of two distinct strains of poliovirus. They also confirmed that monkeys who were infected with one strain and survived were not immune when infected by the second strain. Their finding implied that, to be effective, any vaccine would have to protect against all strains of the virus. While scientists now knew there were at least two distinct strains, they did not know how many strains actually existed in total (Paul, 1971, pp. 224–231).

The effort to learn how many strains of polio there were continued into the 1940s, with funding provided by the newly established National Foundation for Infantile Paralysis (NFIP). In 1948, the NFIP funded a typing program at several university laboratories to determine how many strains or types of polio existed. They supported researchers at the Johns Hopkins University, the University of Utah, the University of Pittsburgh, the University of Kansas, and the University of California, Los Angeles. The work was dull and repetitive but absolutely necessary to any future vaccine. Ultimately, the laboratories tested 196 different samples and found only three strains, one more than Burnet and Macnamara had found in 1931. Of their 196 examples, 82.1% were Type I, 10.2 percent were Type II, and only 7.7 percent were Type III. While the work was done in the individual laboratories, the coordination and funding provided by the NFIP was also crucial to the success of the typing program (Paul, 1971, pp. 232–235).

THE FIRST, AND UNSUCCESSFUL, POLIO VACCINES

Very early in the modern history of poliomyelitis doctors realized that a single attack of polio could confer immunity to the individual. A child who had paralytic polio seldom had another case of the disease. Once the poliovirus was identified, scientists realized that it might be possible to develop a vaccine to confer immunity. This task, however, proved to be immensely challenging and would take scientists almost fifty years of research and testing before Jonas Salk succeeded in the mid-1950s.

Most of the early experimental work on a polio vaccine was done with monkeys, already the common laboratory animal for polio research. If scientists could produce a vaccine that would protect monkeys from subsequent infections of the virus, they might then be able to construct a human vaccine along similar lines. Simon Flexner was among the scientists who worked on artificially stimulating an immune response in monkeys using vaccines. However, although his efforts before 1920 produced some success, the vaccines did not have the kind of consistency and safety necessary to attempt a trial in humans. Researchers debated which kind of vaccine would be best: a killed-virus vaccine or a live-virus vaccine that had been weakened sufficiently so as not to cause a case of polio but would still be capable of producing an immune response strong enough to protect against future infections. Scientists used a variety of methods to kill or weaken the virus. One of the chemicals used was formalin, although the German scientists who tried it initially were not successful. Interestingly, this was the chemical that Dr. Jonas Salk later used to produce his killed-virus vaccine. These early experiments that attempted to develop a monkey vaccine only demonstrated how difficult it would be to develop a polio vaccine for humans. It was not until the 1930s that two physicians would attempt to create a human polio vaccine, an attempt that had unfortunate results.

Dr. Maurice Brodie, a Canadian-born researcher working in New York City, first attempted polio vaccine trials in humans. He used formalin to inactivate the poliovirus in an emulsion of ground-up, infected monkey spinal cord. He first succeeded in immunizing twenty monkeys. He then tried the vaccine on adult volunteers and showed that their immunizing antibodies rose following the injection. Since these volunteers were likely already immune due to previous exposure to wild poliovirus, this initial inoculation was not particularly risky. However, he then proceeded to inoculate twelve children aged between one and six. Brodie was pleased that all showed a rise in their antibody response and that there were no complications. Over the next eight months Brodie and his colleague, Dr. H. W. Park of the New York City Health Laboratory, inoculated some 3,000 children with the vaccine. What exactly happened during this trial is not clear. However, the Brodie vaccine was never again used after this 1935 trial (Paul, 1971, pp. 254–256).

At the same time that Dr. Brodie was developing his vaccine, Dr. John A. Kolmer in Philadelphia worked on a rival vaccine. Dr. Kolmer had begun work on his polio vaccine following a serious polio epidemic in Philadelphia in 1932. Unlike Brodie, who used a killed-virus vaccine, Kolmer decided to use a live but attenuated-virus vaccine. This was a poliovirus weak enough not to cause a case of polio but strong enough to induce the body to produce protective antibodies. The key to such a vaccine, of course, was finding the precise point of attenuation where the vaccine would be both safe and effective. He used a strain of poliovirus that he believed had been weakened by successive passages through various generations of monkeys and then subjected to various chemicals to weaken it further. Kolmer initially tried the vaccine on forty-two monkeys, two adults (including himself), his two children, and twenty-two other children. It seemed to be both safe and effective in these very limited trials. In 1935, Kolmer distributed the vaccine to a number of physicians for trial and they inoculated several thousand children. The results were a disaster. A number of children came down with polio subsequent to their inoculation with the Kolmer vaccine and several of them died of the disease. The trial was quickly ended (Paul, 1971, pp. 256–259).

The failures of Brodie and Kolmer had serious consequences for polio research for the next two decades. Their failures made it clear that researchers did not yet know enough about the poliovirus and how it operated in the human body to design a safe and effective vaccine. Before researchers undertook any future large-scale human test of a polio vaccine, they would need to successfully demonstrate the success of their vaccine in a much larger group of laboratory animals. The size of Brodie's and Kolmer's animal studies were simply too small to obtain any statistically significant results. The fear of causing paralytic polio by trying to inoculate someone against the disease haunted everyone who considered developing a polio vaccine in the 1940s and 1950s. It is interesting to note that while Brodie's and Kolmer's professional colleagues criticized the way they conducted their trials, the U.S. government exercised no oversight over activities of either scientist. It was not until much later that the government set standards for clinical trials such as these.

In spite of the failures of the Brodie and Kolmer vaccines, polio researchers had made significant progress in understanding the disease during the 1930s. They now understood that minor illnesses were an important factor in the spread of the disease during an epidemic and that a significant number of the people infected with the poliovirus would show no obvious symptoms. It was also becoming increasingly clear that the paralytic cases were only a small fraction of the total cases. In addition, there was growing evidence that under normal conditions the poliovirus entered the body through the mouth, not the nose. Scientists could infect monkeys with polio by injecting the nerves of their nasal passages, but an increasing number of polio researchers were convinced that method worked only in the laboratory and not out in the world where people were infected. The mouth as portal of entry for the virus also made sense with the rediscovery of poliovirus in stool samples taken from polio patients and members of their families. Increasingly, doctors regarded polio as an intestinal disease that in a small portion of cases invaded the spinal cord, where it did its damage and caused paralysis. Finally, researchers in Australia and the United States identified two different strains of polio to be followed by a third strain discovered in the 1940s. As the ill-fated vaccine trials of 1935 demonstrated, doctors were nowhere near developing a safe and effective vaccine in the 1930s, but the discoveries they did make proved to be significant in the subsequent successful development of vaccines in the 1950s.

6

The March of Dimes and the Campaign against Polio

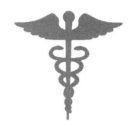

Polio rehabilitation was expensive. When Franklin Roosevelt purchased Warm Springs in 1926 for nearly $200,000, he had given little thought to how he would finance a polio rehabilitation facility. Roosevelt had spent most of his personal fortune purchasing the old resort, and he and his advisors quickly realized that they needed to raise additional funds if Warm Springs was to survive and fulfill FDR's vision of creating a different kind of place for polio rehabilitation. The effort to finance Warm Springs ultimately led to the establishment of the National Foundation for Infantile Paralysis (NFIP), or, as it was more familiarly known, the March of Dimes, perhaps the most successful example of medical philanthropy in the twentieth century.

WARM SPRINGS AND THE PRESIDENT'S BIRTHDAY BALLS

When Roosevelt purchased the Meriwether Inn in 1926 with the intention of turning the failing resort into a first-class polio treatment center, he did not have a clear idea of how he was going to finance this transition or the ongoing expenses of Warm Springs. At the suggestion of Basil O'Connor, Roosevelt's law partner, FDR established the Georgia Warm Springs Foundation to run the facility as a charity and to raise funds in support of its mission of polio rehabilitation. Establishing the foundation also enabled Roosevelt to separate his own money from that of Warm Springs and to accept tax-free gifts to support the rehabilitation of polio patients. Much work needed to be done to transform the resort. The grounds and the buildings needed to be made accessible through the construction of ramps and paved walks. Treatment rooms had to be constructed and new therapy pools built to take advantage of the warm spring waters. Rooms to house and feed the patients had to be remodeled or constructed. In the late 1920s, Warm Springs charged $42 per week for treatment, use of the pools, room and board, and assistance in getting to and from the treatment pools. This sum barely covered current costs, and not everyone who came could pay the full amount. Roosevelt and O'Connor quickly realized that they needed to raise additional funds if Roosevelt's vision was to become a reality (Goldberg, 1981, p. 102).

Roosevelt initially approached some of his wealthy friends to contribute to Warm Springs. For example, Edsel Ford gave $25,000, which was used to construct an enclosed and heated swimming pool so that rehabilitation could continue during the winter. Other friends contributed some $12,000, but that would not be enough to renovate the resort or to help defray the cost of those patients unable to afford the full cost of treatment. A more aggressive program of fundraising was necessary for Warm Springs to succeed.

In 1928, Roosevelt ran for governor of New York. After a spirited campaign, he won the first of his two terms as governor. FDR's political success brought additional national attention to Warm Springs, but it also meant that he had far less time to devote to his favorite non-political project. He asked Basil O'Connor to replace him at the head of the Georgia Warm Springs Foundation. O'Connor had no particular interest in polio or polio rehabilitation, but he was loyal to Roosevelt, and he reluctantly agreed to take charge at the foundation. In spite of his initial reservations, O'Connor quickly threw himself into trying to solve the financial problems facing Warm Springs and soon became committed to the cause of finding a cure or preventive for the disease.

In spite of careful management, Warm Springs ran up substantial operating deficits in the late 1920s and early 1930s. In addition, following the stock market crash in 1929 and the subsequent onset of the Great Depression, charitable giving to the foundation plunged, as it did for charities all across the nation. Donations to Warm Springs fell from $369,000 in 1929 to only $30,000 in 1932, but polio patients still came to Georgia seeking healing, and renovations continued on the facilities (Oshinsky, 2005, p. 47). O'Connor hired Keith Morgan, a New York insurance salesman, to revitalize fundraising and to promote Warm Springs to wealthy potential donors. O'Connor and Morgan quickly realized that the economic crash required them to take a new approach, as even the wealthy closed their wallets to charitable appeals.

Keith Morgan recruited a friend to help rethink and revitalize the fundraising efforts for Warm Springs. Carl Byoir was a public relations man with a flair for selling a wide range of products. At a meeting held in late 1933 to generate new ideas, Byoir suggested that they hold parties throughout the nation to celebrate Roosevelt's birthday and to raise funds for Warm Springs. Roosevelt was president of the United States by this time, and Morgan needed his approval to proceed. When consulted, FDR enthusiastically agreed.

The first Birthday Balls were scheduled for January 29, 1934, and Byoir had only a few months to organize them across the country. Byoir and his associates chose "We Dance So That Others Might Walk" as the slogan for the festivities (Oshinsky, 2005, p. 49). Byoir recruited newspaper publishers, postmasters, and Democratic Party officials to organize Birthday Balls in as many locations as possible. In early January, over 3,000 committees had been established, but Byoir wanted still more. He urged organizers to provide different kinds of balls, including black-tie affairs for the wealthy and dances in union halls for workers. He wanted to include as many people as possible. On January 29, 1934, over 6,000 different dances and parties were held to celebrate Roosevelt's birthday and raise money for Warm Springs and polio rehabilitation. FDR celebrated the occasion by declaring on national radio, "This is the happiest birthday I have ever known" (Oshinsky, 2005, p. 50). O'Connor had hoped that the effort would raise at least $100,000, but on May 9, 1934, after all the monies were counted and the bills paid, the organizing committee gave Roosevelt a check for $1,016,443 (Oshinsky, 2005, p. 50).

As the historian David Oshinsky has noted, the Birthday Balls initiated a wholly new approach to fundraising for charity. Byoir had used "the latest techniques in advertising and public relations to turn traditional philanthropy on its head." Previously, fundraisers had sought a few large gifts, but in the Depression, even the wealthy found it hard to contribute at their traditional rate. Byoir discovered that "the secret lay in small donations." Giving a small amount so that a child could walk again was something almost everybody could do. As Oshinsky has observed, "the key was to reach millions through the modern media—people who had never given to a charity before or who, in truth, had never been asked" (Oshinsky, 2005, p. 51).

Over the next several years, the President's Birthday Ball Commission successfully raised substantial sums. The second ball, in January 1935, brought in over $1.25 million. That year, O'Connor and his associates made an important decision about distributing the money they raised. They decided that 70 percent of the funds raised would remain in the communities that had donated them. This money was allocated to pay for the care of polio patients in their own communities. The other 30 percent went to the President's Birthday Ball Commission to support the Georgia Warm Springs Foundation and to support medical and scientific research on polio. The Commission appointed a small medical advisory committee to make recommendations on the grants to medical researchers. In 1935, the first year the grants were given, the commission awarded sixteen totaling $110,000 (Goldberg, 1981, pp. 156–157). Both decisions set important precedents. When the National Foundation for Infantile Paralysis was established in 1938, it allocated a majority of its funds to the care and rehabilitation of polio patients and another substantial portion to research on the poliovirus, the disease, and a vaccine.

After the success of the 1935 campaign, the Birthday Balls met opposition, and the Commission found it more difficult to raise money. Increasingly, individuals opposed to Roosevelt on political grounds or to his New Deal policies to end the Depression were unwilling to contribute to the effort against polio so long as it was so closely identified with the president. In September 1937, after meeting with O'Connor and other advisors, Roosevelt announced that a new and independent National Foundation for Infantile Paralysis (NFIP) would be established on January 1, 1938, to provide care for polio patients and to fund research and develop a vaccine. Basil O'Connor was appointed director of the NFIP and led it until his death in 1962. Roosevelt would always be identified with the National Foundation, however, and he gave it his full support until his death in 1945. This new organization effectively de-politicized the campaign against polio, and the NFIP went on to become the most effective medical philanthropy in the twentieth century (Oshinsky, 2005, pp. 52–53).

ORGANIZING THE NATIONAL FOUNDATION FOR INFANTILE PARALYSIS

O'Connor faced serious challenges as he gave shape to the new organization in 1938. He rented offices in New York City and began to create committees and advisory boards to help him raise and disburse funds. The most immediate need was to raise money to pay the start-up costs of the organization and to continue the anti-polio campaign begun so effectively by the President's Birthday Ball Commission. O'Connor turned for assistance to Hollywood, where many of the celebrities were sympathetic to Roosevelt's liberal politics. One of Roosevelt's strongest Hollywood supporters was the comedian, actor, and singer Eddie Cantor. In the mid-1930s, Cantor was one of the most popular entertainers, starring in Hollywood musicals and hosting a popular weekly radio show. During a brainstorming session with his entertainment friends, Cantor suggested calling the 1938 campaign the "March of Dimes." This was a play on the popular "March of Time" newsreels that brought the world's news to moviegoers before they saw the main feature. Cantor proposed asking people to send their dimes directly to Roosevelt at the White House. In spite of a possible political backlash, Roosevelt agreed to the scheme. Cantor used his weekly radio show to announce the program and its slogan and to urge Americans to send in their dimes, or whatever they could, to FDR to help support this new campaign against polio. Cantor declared, "The March of Dimes will enable all persons, even the children, to show our president we are with him in this battle" (Oshinsky, 2005, p. 54). Other Hollywood celebrities, including The Lone Ranger, Jack Benny, Bing Crosby, and Rudy Vallee, joined Cantor in appealing to their fans to contribute to the fight against polio. The White House was warned to expect some increase in mail, but they were overwhelmed by the national response. The White House normally received around 5,000 pieces of mail daily. On the third day of the March of Dimes campaign, they received 150,000 letters containing dimes and other coins and currency. By the time the campaign came to a close, the White House had received 2,680,000 dimes ($286,000) as well as additional money and checks. Including money not sent to the White House, the NFIP raised $1.8 million in 1938, substantially exceeding the best year of the Birthday Balls. Not surprisingly, the success of the 1938 campaign and the popularity of the slogan led the NFIP to call their fundraising branch the March of Dimes (Oshinsky, 2005, pp. 54–55; Smith, 1990, p. 75).

Basil O'Connor tightly controlled the National Foundation during his many years as its director. O'Connor and his handpicked associates at the national office in New York established policy and ensured that the local chapters complied. There were salaried officials at both the national and local levels, but there were also many volunteers, especially in the fundraising arm of the organization. The salaried staff addressed the needs of local polio patients and disbursed monies to families, hospitals, and other institutions to pay for polio care. Most of the volunteers participated for a brief time every year in the annual March of Dimes campaign to raise funds to support the work of the NFIP. Half of the money raised went to the National Foundation to support its operations and to fund scientific research and some polio care, especially complicated and expensive respiratory care. The other half of the money stayed in the local community to pay for the care of local residents who had contracted polio. This aspect of the March of Dimes campaigns helped make them so popular (Oshinsky, 2005, pp. 64–65).

THE MARCH OF DIMES

From the very beginning, raising money was a central focus of the National Foundation. Without the money brought in by the March of Dimes, none of the other activities would have been possible. There would have been no aid to polio patients and their families, and no money for the scientific grants to medical researchers that ultimately led to two successful vaccines. In the earliest years of the organization, O'Connor and his associates faced major challenges to raising substantial sums of money.

In 1938, when the NFIP was organized, the Great Depression left many Americans with few spare dimes to contribute. With the rise in defense spending in the early 1940s, the Depression finally ended as the country went back to work, but now the war against Germany and Japan seemed to take priority over the war on polio. Roosevelt, however, wanted no holding back in the campaign against polio during World War II, in spite of other demands on the nation's resources. He wrote O'Connor, "The fight being waged against infantile paralysis . . . is an essential part of the struggle in which we are all engaged. . . . To me it is one of the front lines of our National Defense" (Oshinsky, 2005, p. 68).

The March of Dimes introduced several new techniques to encourage American support for the campaign against polio. The Birthday Balls continued in some communities, but the March of Dimes also developed many other ways to raise money. Drawing on the important precedent of the Birthday Balls, O'Connor pursued the strategy of raising large sums of money in small donations from millions of contributors. In the 1940s, the National Foundation drew upon its friends in Hollywood and produced several short films that showed in movie theaters before the main feature. When these were shown, a March of Dimes volunteer or the theater's ushers would seek contributions by passing through the theater with a bucket. In 1941, the March of Dimes collected $435,000 in movie theaters. The theater collections became a major source of NFIP revenue during the war years. These collections helped fuel the rapid rise in March of Dimes contributions from $1.8 million in 1938 to $19 million in 1945. About $8 million of the 1945 revenues came from contributions in the theater collection boxes (Oshinsky, 2005, pp. 68–69).

The end of World War II and Roosevelt's death in 1945 forced the March of Dimes to rethink and reorganize its fundraising activities. In 1946, the movie studios ended collections in the theaters they owned in favor of a $30,000 contribution to the March of Dimes (Oshinsky, 2005, p. 80). This significant loss of revenue for the NFIP came at a time when the number of polio cases needing assistance was increasing and when the accelerated pace of

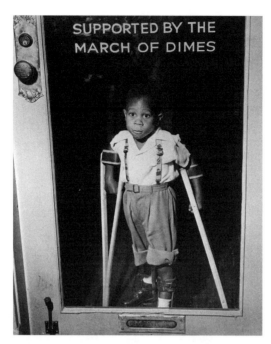

A child in 1951 wearing braces and using crutches provided through the fundraising efforts of the March of Dimes. (March of Dimes)

scientific research put additional demands on the organization's finances. Without the movie house revenue, the March of Dimes had to look elsewhere for the necessary funds.

The same year that revenue from the movie houses dried up, the March of Dimes introduced its first poster child. They took a good-looking young boy or girl showing obvious signs of having had polio, such as using a wheelchair or wearing braces, and made him or her the official representative of that year's fundraising campaign. They hoped to inspire pity for the crippled child and thereby encourage contributions to the March of Dimes. The posters asked people to contribute to help pay for the care of children crippled by the disease and to give so that research could find a vaccine that would prevent any more children from becoming crippled. Since polio rates were rising in the United States, this was a powerful image. It was also a controversial one, for it exploited the young patients by putting them on display to raise money for the cause. Donald Anderson was the first national poster child in 1946, and every year thereafter the NFIP chose one or more national poster children to represent the campaign. Many local chapters also selected local poster

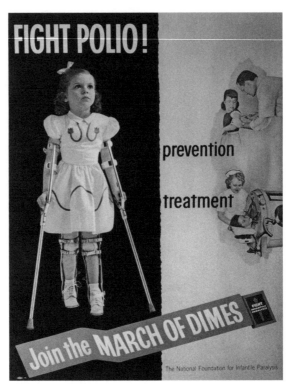

The March of Dimes Poster for 1955 with poster child Mary Kosloski. (March of Dimes)

children to help with publicity for the annual March of Dimes campaign (Oshinsky, 2005, pp. 81–83). The poster children often had conflicted feelings about being put on display, even for a good cause. Some, like Carol Boyer, remember feeling "very special," and that "it was fun, but it also made you feel like you have to look perfect" (Seavey, 1998, pp. 78–79). Kathy Vastyshak was never a poster child, but, because her father volunteered for the March of Dimes, her picture often appeared in the local newspaper during the annual appeal for funds. She recalls that she never liked the attention: "I always thought it made me different" (Vastyshak, 2002, interview). The poster child idea, however, proved to be a successful innovation and was copied by many later medical philanthropies.

The March of Dimes had a Public Relations Department that was adept at stoking the public's fear of polio and its awareness of the NFIP campaign against the disease. The poster child was only one piece of a multifaceted effort. The Public Relations Department sent out a steady stream of news releases and articles prepared for publication in local and national magazines and newspapers. Many of these articles offered advice on how to avoid polio, especially during summer when the polio epidemics were most likely to occur. They warned parents not to let their children near swimming pools or swimming holes, to keep them from drinking at public water fountains, and to stay away from crowded places like movie theaters. They also publicized the warning signs of polio, including a stiff neck, the inability to touch one's chin to one's chest, and muscle pain and weakness. There were also news releases touting the latest scientific discovery about the disease that had been funded with March of Dimes contributions. There were human-interest stories about how individuals and families were successfully coping with polio, invariably with the assistance of the NFIP. And there were always more appeals for money to assist polio victims and to pursue the search for a vaccine.

The March of Dimes also developed the new strategy of house-to-house solicitation beginning in the late 1940s. In 1950, the March of Dimes chapter in Maricopa County, Arizona, which included Phoenix, tried a new approach to solicitation. At 7:00 p.m. on January 16, mothers throughout the city and county took to the sidewalks to call on their neighbors to contribute to the campaign against polio. City authorities cooperated by operating fire and police sirens. Advertisements had previously appeared in newspapers, and posters announcing the march had been placed in store windows. Children in schools were reminded to encourage their parents to participate. Individuals and families willing to give to the March of Dimes were told to turn on their porch lights as a welcome sign to the volunteers collecting funds. Over 2,300 volunteers, many of them mothers, collected $44,890 from 42,288 donors in one hour. This successful local campaign became known as the Mothers' March on Polio and quickly became a model for other communities across the nation (Oshinsky, 2005, pp. 87–88).

The success of the Phoenix effort led the NFIP to begin to plan for 1951, when they tried to replicate the Mothers' March on Polio in communities throughout the country. The national office of the NFIP developed and sent to each chapter detailed plans for the Mothers' March. Well before the January date, the Public Relations Department worked tirelessly to publicize the event and to encourage both the volunteers who would collect the funds and the families who would contribute. Again, as in Phoenix, a lit porch light signaled a welcome to the marching mothers. Mothers across the nation joined the March because the time commitment was minimal—one hour marching and perhaps another one or two turning in the funds collected—and it made them participants in the campaign against polio. Many mothers knew someone who had been stricken by the disease, and all mothers fervently hoped that the NFIP would find a cure for polio before it struck their own children.

Between 1951 and 1955, the March of Dimes raised $250 million, much of that from the Mothers' March. It quickly became the largest source of funds for the National Foundation (Oshinsky, 2005, pp. 88–90).

The March of Dimes became the most successful medical charity in the middle of the twentieth century because it was well organized and run, because it was willing to innovate with fundraising techniques, and because it had a powerful message that appealed to parents and others. Basil O'Connor was a superb chief executive completely dedicated to ending the scourge of polio by any legitimate means. He and his associates were willing to try almost anything to raise the necessary funds—Birthday Balls, poster children, collections in movie theaters, support from Hollywood celebrities, and marching mothers. If a local chapter, like the one in Phoenix, discovered a new way to raise funds, the NFIP took the approach and applied it nationally. Finally, the appeal of the March of Dimes was a powerful one, especially in the peaceful years following World War II. Millions of veterans had come home from the war wanting nothing more than to marry their sweethearts, have children, and raise them in one of the many new suburbs springing up around major cities. Polio threatened to destroy that post-war American dream. No parent wanted a child encased in heavy leather and steel braces, dependent on a wheelchair for mobility, or, even worse, confined to an iron lung. By volunteering for a few hours every January or contributing their dimes and dollars, Americans felt they were participating in the national campaign to make childhood safe once again.

AIDING FAMILIES

Polio was an expensive disease. It was expensive to treat a case of polio and to rehabilitate the polio patient. Scientific research was also expensive, and when a vaccine was ready to be tested, setting up a nationwide test cost the NFIP millions of dollars. From 1938 to 1959 the March of Dimes raised over $622 million. In that same time period, the National Foundation spent over $315 million on aid to polio patients and their families for hospital expenses, for the cost of rehabilitation, and for equipment such as braces, crutches, and wheelchairs. Over 315,000 polio patients were assisted during the 1940s and 1950s. In addition to aiding patients, the NFIP spent an additional $55 million on scientific and medical research and another $33 million on educating and training medical professionals such as physicians, physical therapists, nurses, and respiratory therapists to care for polio patients (Carter, 1961, pp. 95–96).

Polio patients and their families were particularly grateful for the financial assistance from the National Foundation. In the 1940s and 1950s, few families had medical or hospital insurance to cover the cost of polio care. In 1939, only 6 percent of families had medical insurance, and while that number would rise to 24 percent in 1945, many families could not afford the high cost of caring for a polio patient. The average cost of a case of polio in these years was between $2000 and $3000, depending on the severity of the case. If the patient needed an iron lung, the cost could rise to $10,000 a year. Some families were especially hard hit when the breadwinner, usually the husband in these years, came down with polio. Then, the cost of polio was compounded by the loss of income when he could not work. The median annual wage in 1940 was $877, and only 3.7 percent of the population earned more than $3,000. Clearly, most families could not easily pay the cost of a serious case of polio (Wilson, 1998, p. 483).

Local chapters of the National Foundation for Infantile Paralysis retained about 50 percent of the money collected in the community by the March of Dimes and made decisions about who received aid. Doctors and hospitals were required to report cases of polio to the public health authorities, and in many communities, these officials also sent the names of new victims to the local NFIP chapter. Typically, the chairman of the chapter would send a letter to the patient's family informing them of the National Foundation's readiness to help with expenses. The chapter invited families to meet with local officials to discuss their needs. After taking information from the new polio families, the executive committee of the chapter determined how much aid to provide. The national NFIP office provided some general guidelines to assist local officials in making their decisions, but there were no rigid criteria to qualify for aid. Local chapters had considerable discretion to make decisions appropriate to the need of the families, the resources available, and the standards of the community. The goal was to provide the best possible care without requiring the family to take on an undue financial burden or lower its standard of living. Families who could afford it were expected to contribute to the expense of care, but the NFIP tried to cover those costs that would mean a financial hardship to the family. The local chapters did not make decisions about what kind of care was necessary or appropriate; that was for the physicians to decide. The NFIP tried to make the recommended care possible. Not every family qualified for aid from the NFIP, although 75–80 to eighty percent of polio families received some assistance (Sills, 1957, pp. 132–134).

One of the challenges facing the March of Dimes in paying for polio care was that rehabilitation often stretched into months and even years. Each chapter had to budget not only for that year's new cases but also for the polio patients from previous years who were still undergoing rehabilitation, who still needed surgery to correct deformities, or who needed new braces and wheelchairs. A serious epidemic could severely strain the budget of even well-funded chapters. The National Foundation did maintain an emergency fund to assist local chapters facing an immediate crisis, but some chapters were forced to make an emergency appeal during the year to supplement funds raised by the Mothers' March in January (Sills, 1957, pp. 135–136). Increasingly, the national office of the NFIP took on the very expensive care for patients dependent on iron lungs. In November 1950, there were 583 patients who relied on an iron lung to breathe. These patients often required around-the-clock specialized nursing care, and even when they went home in their iron lungs, the expenses of such patients were beyond the financial ability of most families. By the 1950s, the NFIP established fifteen respirator centers around the country to care for iron lung patients. This enabled them to reduce costs and to provide better care, although it was still very expensive (Rothman, 1997, pp. 63–64).

SUPPORTING RESEARCH AND EDUCATION

When the National Foundation for Infantile Paralysis began operating in 1938, there were almost no sources of funding to support research on poliomyelitis and to develop a vaccine. The President's Birthday Ball Commission had initiated a research program, but it had been in operation for only a few years and had awarded relatively few grants. Unlike today, when the U.S. government is a major supporter of scientific and medical research, in the late 1930s, the government provided almost no support to polio research or any other kind of medical research. From 1938 to 1962, the National Foundation was the major source of funds to support research on the disease and to educate health care professionals in the care and treatment of polio patients. During those years the organization spent $69 million on research, about 11 percent of the total funds raised by the March of Dimes. The NFIP spent another $50 million (8 percent) of the funds on education during the polio epidemics (Paul, 1971, p. 312).

The money provided by the March of Dimes proved essential to the conquest of polio. In 1938, there were fewer than fifty virologists studying viruses in the United States, and only a small number were interested in polio. The NFIP grants helped fund an expansion in the number of virologists and basic research into the nature of viruses as well as increased direct research on the poliovirus. This new and generous source of funds had an immediate impact on polio researchers. Dr. John Paul, a polio researcher at Yale University, described it as like "the sudden appearance of a fairy godmother of quite mammoth proportions who thrived on publicity" (Paul, 1971, p. 311). The research program funded by the March of Dimes will be discussed in detail in Chapter 9, but it is important to note that unraveling the mysteries of the poliovirus and developing a vaccine would have been substantially delayed without this funding.

In addition to supporting scientific research, the NFIP also paid to train thousands of health professionals in polio care and treatment. This was particularly important in the 1940s and 1950s as the epidemics increased in size and severity. The Foundation funded the training of nearly 300 physicians, almost 2,700 physical therapists, over 700 medical social workers, and several thousand other professionals involved in polio care and treatment (Carter, 1961, p. 96). In addition, the NFIP often used its funds to send doctors, nurses, and therapists to communities experiencing an epidemic. An epidemic could quickly overwhelm local medical resources, and the National Foundation often paid physicians, nurses, and therapists to travel to the location of the epidemic to relieve the local staff.

CONCLUSION

The National Foundation for Infantile Paralysis and the March of Dimes revolutionized medical charitable giving and advocacy for a specific disease during their long and ultimately successful campaign against polio. Starting with the President's Birthday Balls, Basil O'Connor and his associates were innovators in the methods of raising money. Their first important decision, necessitated in part by the economic conditions of the Depression, was to seek a large number of small contributions rather than a few large contributions as had been the previous practice of medical philanthropies. Having made that decision, they thought up new ways to inform the public about polio and to induce them to contribute their dimes and dollars: dancing on Roosevelt's birthday, filling buckets with change in movie theaters, securing the endorsement of Hollywood celebrities and prominent politicians, having mothers march through neighborhoods accepting contributions on lighted porches, and advertising the cause through poster children. While the March of Dimes developed new strategies to raise money, the National Foundation found innovative ways to spend it. Half of the money raised stayed in the local community to provide financial assistance to families for doctors' bills, hospital care, rehabilitation, and necessary assistive devices. Part of the other half funded almost all of the scientific and medical research that developed new techniques in virology, discovered how polio was spread in the community, identified the three types of polio, and, most importantly, created two effective polio vaccines. In addition, the national funds supported the training of thousands of health professionals in the care and treatment of polio patients. Finally, of course, these funds paid the expenses of running the organization and raising the money. In all of these areas, the National Foundation for Infantile Paralysis and the March of Dimes established a new model that many subsequent medical charities followed.

7

Summers of Fear: Acute Polio

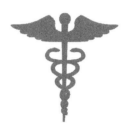

"I'm afraid it's polio." Every parent dreaded hearing those words during the height of the polio epidemics in the 1940s and 1950s. They meant that another child, or sometimes a teenager or even an adult, had been diagnosed with polio. Once the diagnosis was pronounced, the child was quickly introduced to a world of hospitals, doctors, and isolation from family and friends. Most polio patients in these years were cared for in special polio hospitals or in isolation wards of general hospitals during the acute phase of the illness, when they were sickest and most likely to transmit the disease to someone else. Polio is a very painful disease in the acute phase as the poliovirus damages and destroys nerves in the spinal cord, thereby paralyzing the muscles that enable us to move. Doctors could do little once the virus reached the spinal cord other than to try to keep the patient comfortable and hope that the permanent damage would be minimal. Once the acute phase passed, usually in ten days to two weeks, the patients were sent to rehabilitation to try to rebuild muscles that had only been weakened and to learn to compensate for the muscles that had been destroyed. Rehabilitation could be as short as a few weeks or as long as two years or more, depending on the damage done by the poliovirus. Rehabilitation provided the polio survivors with the new skills and equipment they needed to return to school and work, to return to living as normal a life as possible.

"I'M AFRAID IT'S POLIO": THE DIAGNOSIS OF POLIO

Polio was the most feared childhood disease in the mid-twentieth century. Parents feared it for several reasons. Polio was capricious. No one knew when or where the next epidemic would occur. In an epidemic, no one, not even the doctors, could predict who would come down with polio, or how severe it would be for those who contracted the disease. And once polio struck, there was nothing the physicians could do to stop the spread of paralysis; the virus had to run its course while the doctors kept the patient comfortable. The sociologist Fred Davis has written that statistics about the rate of polio "cannot account for the awe and dread" with which Americans regarded the disease. He thought polio's capacity to permanently cripple young children inspired much of the dread of the disease, but in fact that wasn't sufficient to explain the widespread fear. By the post–World War II period, polio "had emerged in popular thought as more than a sometimes crippling disease of children: it was regarded as a powerful symbol of blind, devastating, and uncontrollable misfortune whose victims were specially entitled to the support and good will of the community" (Davis, 1991, pp. 6–7). One father whose son had polio felt that the disease shattered the American dream: "Polio kills that. It kills that dream. It cuts it short" (Davis, 1991, p. 41).

Brenda Serotte was only eight when she came down with polio in 1954, but she remembers how polio was one of the subjects that adults talked about in hushed voices: "Of all the topics, when the women spoke of polio their voices lowered an octave. This, I gathered, was worse than the Bomb or Communism" (Serotte, 2006, p. 71). During the summer of 1954, when polio fears were especially high, Brenda's parents gave her a "whole new set of rules and warnings: Don't dare drink from a public water fountain in any park, at school, or when visiting the zoo. Be sure to sit at least one seat apart in the movies, and never share popcorn. If the theater gets overcrowded, it will get hot, and then you have to come home. Do not put even your big toe into a public wading pool and don't play with anyone, not *anyone*, who sneezes" (Serotte, 2006, p. 71). She remembers hearing adults say that "polio's worst curse wasn't death. It was confinement and deformity. *Confined to a wheelchair. Locked into braces. He will walk with braces and crutches for the rest of his life*" (Serotte, 2006, pp. 71–72). In spite of her mother's warnings, warnings that were repeated by mothers across the country, Brenda came down with polio shortly after Labor Day.

Part of the fear of polio derived from the fact that the symptoms in its early stages were like those of many other diseases, many of them minor. In these years, whenever a child became sick, especially in the summer, parents worried that it might be polio. Polio begins innocently enough with a fever, a feeling of fatigue, and perhaps an upset stomach. But many diseases begin that way, and until paralysis appeared, or a special test called a spinal tap was performed in the hospital, even doctors found it difficult to diagnose polio. Doctors made house calls in the polio years, but many parents were reluctant to call the doctor unless they were sure their child was seriously ill. Most families did not have health insurance, and there was no point in calling the doctor for the many minor illnesses of childhood. Arvid Schwartz developed polio in western Minnesota in 1952 when he was twelve. He recalls falling off his bike, which was unusual for him. A few days later, he woke up feeling that he had "this flu." When the illness persisted for a day or two, his parents finally called the doctor, who drove out to their farm to see him. He remembers that "in 1952 in rural Minnesota you didn't go to the doctor the minute you ran a fever. You waited until you were sure something was wrong" (Seavey, 1998, p. 253). The doctor diagnosed the illness as "some kind of flu." Three days after the doctor's visit, Arvid tried to get out of bed in the morning and fell to the floor. His parents again called the doctor, who made another visit to the farm. Only on this second visit did he suspect polio and recommend that Arvid's parents take him to a hospital in Minneapolis, several hours away by car (Sass, 1996, pp. 143–144).

The March of Dimes widely publicized the warning signs of polio. These signs included a sore throat, swallowing difficulty, sore muscles, a fever, an upset stomach, a headache, and a stiff neck. These were fairly common symptoms for a variety of ailments, so deciding whether they were warning signs of polio was often difficult for parents and doctors alike. One common test was asking a child to touch her chin to her chest, something most children could easily do. The stiff neck that often accompanied early-stage polio made this impossible. Many parents had their children perform the test every day during polio season. The mother of Linda Atkins insisted on the daily test as "constant proof that her children were still healthy—safe from the death moving all around us." That worked all summer until one day when Linda could no longer pass. The doctor soon diagnosed her with polio and sent her to the hospital (Wilson, 2005, p. 21).

Teenagers and adults coming down with polio often tried to fight off the symptoms and to continue with their school and work responsibilities. For example, Hugh Gallagher was a student at Haverford College in Pennsylvania when he developed the symptoms of a bad cold. He kept getting worse and developed severe pains in his back and a stiff neck. Gallagher tried to register for classes and carry on normally, but the increasing pain made it difficult to do anything, including sleeping. When he finally saw the college physician, the doctor urged him to go to the infirmary, but Gallagher refused, as his parents were arriving that night for parents' weekend. By the time his family arrived he felt no better, and they walked him across campus to the infirmary. The next morning Gallagher discovered to his dismay that paralysis was beginning to creep up his leg. The nurse called the doctor, who said to send Gallagher to the hospital as quickly as possible. Both of his legs were paralyzed by the time the ambulance arrived to take him to a hospital in Philadelphia (Gallagher, 1998, pp. 19–24).

Bea Wright was a single mother with three boys. She worked at the local National Foundation for Infantile Paralysis office in Detroit. Wright was at work when she began to feel ill. Initially, she thought she was coming down with the flu. Throughout the day, she felt worse and worse, and the pain increased. In the afternoon she told her staff, "Look, I don't want to be an alarmist, but I have every symptom of polio." Her staff downplayed the notion and suggested that working with polio patients had made her imagine that she was developing polio. The next day she found getting up for work very difficult. Hurrying to catch the bus, she fell. Wright managed to keep a previously scheduled breakfast meeting. Later in the day, she was at a hospital to oversee a photographer taking pictures of children helped by the March of Dimes. Since she felt so ill, she was examined by a doctor who diagnosed her ailment as polio. The photo session was immediately cancelled and Wright was quickly admitted to the hospital as a polio patient (Chappell, 1960, pp. 12–13, 17–18, 20–22).

Children and even older patients were not always told that they had come down with polio. Doctors in the 1940s and 1950s usually told parents their diagnosis of polio out of the hearing of the sick child. It was the parents' responsibility to tell the child. Some parents told their child the bad news immediately, while others withheld the specific diagnosis, perhaps hoping it wasn't true. Children occasionally overheard the doctor telling their parents they had polio, and children were certainly sensitive to their parents' shocked and worried response to the doctor's diagnosis. Sometimes, even when they were told what had made them sick, children didn't fully realize what they had. Twelve-year-old Richard Owen's parents told him he had "poliomyelitis," but only much later did he realize that he had contracted the same disease as President Roosevelt, "infantile paralysis." Adolescents who had not been told the diagnosis sometimes found ways to learn the name of their illness. Hugh Gallagher's physician wouldn't tell him the diagnosis, but Gallagher suspected he had polio. So when a new physician examined him, Gallagher asked how severe his polio was. His fears were confirmed when this new doctor said they didn't yet know. For all patients, doctors often tried to downplay the severity of the disease by assuring patients that they would soon recover and be fine. But since no physician in these early stages could accurately predict how much paralysis was permanent, patients were sometimes seriously misled. Thirty-year-old Louis Sternburg's physician initially told him that he had a "mild case. Nonparalytic." Unfortunately, Sternburg would be permanently paralyzed from the neck down (Wilson, 2005, pp. 29–30).

Bea Wright was already at the hospital when she was diagnosed with polio, but many polio patients had a harrowing and painful ride to the hospital. Acute polio was very painful, and being bounced around in an ambulance or family car on the way to the hospital was often excruciating. Some patients had to endure only a short trip across town to the hospital accepting polio patients, but patients who lived on farms or in small rural communities often had long and very painful rides to the hospital. Even short rides could hurt. Shirley Paul's father took her to the hospital in Washington, D.C., and though it was a short ride, she repeatedly asked her father, "Daddy, Daddy! Go slower! It hurts!" Every bump and pothole shot pain through her whole body (Wilson, 2005, 37–38). Charlotte Pugleasa felt "every bump, every railroad track" on the sixty-mile ride across Minnesota to the hospital (Wilson, 2005, pp. 37–38).

Parents and ambulance drivers often had to decide where to take the patient, as not all hospitals accepted acute polio patients. Some communities had separate isolation hospitals to care for polio patients and patients with other contagious diseases. In other cities, hospitals had separate wings or separate wards housing up to twenty polio patients. In 1943, Chicago had only seven hospitals that accepted acute polio patients, but by 1956, thirty-five hospitals cared for these patients. Ambulance drivers generally knew where to take polio patients, but parents sometimes had to go to more than one hospital before they found one that would admit their child (Wilson, 2005, pp. 36–37).

African American parents faced an additional challenge in finding a hospital to care for their child. The polio epidemics occurred during the era of Jim Crow segregation in the United States. This was the period when all southern states and some northern ones legally required segregation of the races. Almost all southern hospitals and medical facilities were segregated into those caring for black patients and those caring for white patients. Some northern and western hospitals had separate wards for black and white patients, with the facilities for black patients generally inferior to those for white patients. Some smaller southern towns had only a white hospital, which meant that African American parents had to travel to the closest town with a hospital that would admit their child, and that might be some distance away. Although segregated facilities were supposed to be equal, almost all of the black institutions were inferior in terms of equipment and the training of their staff. Occasionally, as in the 1944 epidemic in Hickory, North Carolina, the magnitude of the epidemic required doctors to break the racial barriers and put black and white patients in adjacent beds; however, as soon as the epidemic began to lessen, the hospital moved the black and white patients into separate wards.

ACUTE POLIO AND THE ISOLATION HOSPITAL

Because polio was highly contagious, ambulance crews and hospital personnel took special care in handling newly diagnosed polio patients. The ambulance crew that took Robert Gurney to the hospital covered his face and entire body with a rubber sheet and a blanket. When his mother asked why, they replied, "Because we don't know if he's contagious, and we don't want to take any chances" (Sass, 1996, p. 22). The male and female ambulance attendants who came for Brenda Serotte were both in white uniforms and wearing masks. They quickly loaded her on the stretcher, covered her face and hair with a sheet, and carried her down the stairs to the ambulance. Serotte recalls that "I tried to blow the sheet off my face because I couldn't breathe right. It made them mad" (Serotte, 2006, p. 68). The ambulance crew that delivered Jane Needham to the hospital in 1949 was not allowed to use the elevator for fear that they would contaminate it. They had to carry her stretcher up the narrow outside fire escape to the second floor polio ward. When the heavy fire door slammed shut, Jane felt cut off "forever from the life that I had known" (Needham, 1959, pp. 52–53).

Most isolation hospitals in this period did not allow visitors to reduce the likelihood of spreading contagious diseases like polio. In most cases, even parents and spouses were not allowed to visit their sick children or spouse once they had been admitted to the isolation hospital or ward. Most hospitals in this period did not have private or semi-private rooms; patients were cared for in large rooms, or wards, of four to twenty beds. The agonizing separation at the door of the polio hospital or ward was very difficult for both the patient and the family members who were kept from accompanying the patient to the ward. Because parents had often downplayed the seriousness of the illness, hoping to reassure their child that he or she would soon be well, children were often unprepared to be hospitalized, let alone "abandoned" by their parents at the hospital door. On the way to the hospital, Charlene Pugleasa begged her mother not to leave her there, in part because she had never before been in a hospital overnight. At the hospital, as Charlene's mother went to accompany her daughter to her room, the nurse told her that she could not go beyond the doors to the polio ward. Charlene remembers crying, "'Mom, please don't leave me here.' And they just swung those doors. My mother's face was in this little window and she was crying. . . . There were no parting, loving, kind words because they whisked me off so fast." As she was wheeled to the polio ward, Charlene recalls "just totally feeling alone in the world" (Seavey, 1998, p. 124).

As we have seen, polio was often hard to diagnose based solely on the early symptoms of the disease. There was, however, a test many hospitals administered that provided a more certain diagnosis, the spinal tap. Tapping into the fluid surrounding the spinal cord required the physician to insert a long needle between the vertebrae of the spine. The physician then withdrew spinal fluid into the syringe. Under a microscope, the pathologist counted the number of cells per cubic millimeter in the fluid. Normal cell counts were 3 to 10 per cubic millimeter. The average case of polio had a cell count of 350, although the range could be from 10 to 700. Higher cell counts meant a more certain diagnosis of polio (Lewin, 1941, pp. 74–76).

Except for the feeling of abandonment, the spinal tap was often the most memorable aspect of admission to a polio hospital. Many doctors used a local anesthetic before inserting the large needle, and a well-done procedure was relatively painless. Doctors, however, were not equally skilled in administering a spinal tap, and many polio patients experienced considerable pain during the procedure. For example, Robert Hudson's spinal tap felt like someone was "driving a wooden stake in my back" (Wilson, 2005, p. 41). For others, the anticipation was worse than the actual tap itself. Charles Mee remembers catching a "glimpse of the needle, which was terrifyingly long; surely they had made some mistake, surely this was a veterinarian's needle, meant for horses." While assistants held him down, the doctor inserted the needle into his spine. Surprisingly, Mee experienced little pain, but there was still "fear, along with the dread of the expected confirmation of polio" (Mee, 1999, p. 15). Typically, once the spinal tap was completed, the patient was taken to the isolation ward.

While intense, the pain of the spinal tap lasted only a short time. The pain of being isolated from parents or spouses when sick with acute polio lasted much longer. While polio patients were sometimes quarantined in their own homes, which meant that no one except doctors and nurses could enter the home or leave, more often in the 1940s and 1950s they were treated in hospitals. Larger cities often had separate isolation hospitals for all contagious diseases, and large hospitals sometimes had a separate isolation wing. Smaller hospitals might have an isolation floor or sometimes only a single ward for contagious patients. Most hospitals established a strict no-visitors policy for as long as the polio patient was in isolation. This meant that parents could not visit their children, and a husband could not visit his wife or a wife her husband. There were two reasons for the policy. Most important, by keeping visitors out of the polio wards, hospitals hoped to limit the spread of polio by preventing visitors from carrying the virus outside the hospital. In addition, caring for acute polio patients in an epidemic was often intense, and allowing no visitors meant that doctors and nurses could more effectively carry out their duties. But what made sense from the hospital's point of view was very difficult from the patient's perspective and that of the family.

Children, even teenagers, were accustomed to having their parents, and especially their mothers, at their bedsides when they were sick. Children now found themselves in this strange place surrounded by other equally sick patients, and attended by nurses and doctors dressed in white with a white mask over their noses and mouths. It was like a nightmare, except that it was real. Charles Mee remembered that "the isolation ward was well named: I have never been so alone in my life as in that bed, where I was confined for the next three weeks, feverish and contagious" (Mee, 1999, p. 16). For Carole Sauer, "the scariest thing about that isolation ward . . . was the separation from my parents. We were allowed no visitors at all" (Sass, 1996, p. 107). Like Sauer, James Berry "was most depressed about the total isolation of the hospital ward. I saw nobody from morning to night except nurses in sterile caps, gowns, and masks" (Sass, 1996, p. 226). Parents and spouses often stood outside the hospital hoping to glimpse their child or spouse through the window, and, if the windows were open, they might even be able to talk to the polio patients confined inside.

Some hospitals did allow parents and spouses to visit, even while patients were in isolation. Boston hospitals during the 1955 epidemic discovered that parents and spouses were willing volunteers in the care of their family members, and that took some of the strain off the nursing staff during this severe epidemic. When I was in isolation, my mother was not allowed to visit me. However, because the hospital was short of staff, she was allowed to volunteer and give hot packs to all the patients on the ward, and, of course, to spend a few minutes with me. Brenda Serotte remembers that her parents were allowed to visit her the first morning in the hospital, but "they came in garbed all in white, including face masks that covered everything except their eyes" (Serotte, 2006, p. 80). Parents and spouses were also admitted when the doctors feared that a patient might die.

In retrospect, many of these no-visiting regulations were unnecessary, and the enforced separation from parents and spouses contributed to the anguish of acute polio. By the late 1940s, scientific research had demonstrated that by the time one family member was hospitalized with polio, all the other members of the family had already been exposed. So, keeping close family members from visiting offered no additional protection to the individuals or to the community. In addition, doctors, nurses, and other hospital personnel who took care of the polio patients were allowed to go home at the end of the day. Many doctors and nurses worried about carrying polio home to their children and spouses, which occasionally happened, but there were generally no restrictions on the movement of hospital personnel. Some hospitals called for volunteers to help care for polio patients during serious epidemics, and again their ability to enter and leave the hospital was not limited. Finally, hospitals that admitted close family members during the acute stage of polio generally found them to be helpful in easing the anxieties of the patients and often useful in helping to care for them. Thus, while the regulations had a certain logic to them, they were unlikely to have been much use in stemming a polio epidemic, and they certainly increased the psychological agony of acute polio.

PARALYSIS AND THE PAIN OF POLIO

One of the most frightening aspects of acute polio was the spread of paralysis across the body. As the virus destroyed or damaged nerves leading to particular muscles, these muscles became paralyzed. Many patients were lucid during the early phase of acute polio and recall how frightened and puzzled they were as parts of their bodies refused to work. Hugh Gallagher first noticed that he could no longer wiggle the toes of his left foot: "I could send the usual message, in the usual way, from my will to my foot—'move'—but there was no movement." He began to try each toe, and as he did he noticed that "the lack of movement seemed to expand its area." As he experimented with trying to move the leg, the paralysis slowly moved up the leg to his hip. He hoped it would stop and even reverse itself, but after a few minutes the paralysis began to expand by creeping down his right leg (Gallagher, 1998, pp. 23–24). When polio attacked fifteen-year-old Irving Zola, he was convinced he was going to die. He recalled that "every time I was conscious enough to appreciate what was going on, another part of my body felt immobilized. When the process finally stopped, I knew I wouldn't die, but almost wished I had. I had little strength. I could only turn my head from side to side and raise my left arm" (Zola, 1983, p. 9).

Many polio survivors remember the last walk they took unaided as the disease began to weaken and paralyze their leg muscles. Irving Zola took his last walk at home before being hospitalized: "I rose weakly from my bed. My legs, however, would not hold me and with a scream for help I collapsed. . . . I was never to walk normally again" (Zola, 1983, p. 9). During his night at the college infirmary, Hugh Gallagher got up to use the bathroom. He managed to "stabilize" his weak legs so he could walk to the bathroom and make it back to bed. Those were his last steps, and as he later observed, "There should have been more ceremony attached to them" (Gallagher, 1998, p. 22). For some, their walk into the hospital was the last one they would take under their own power. David Kangas had been forced to drop out of a parade to benefit the March of Dimes because he was too weak to continue. After the family doctor decided that he probably had polio, Kangas's parents took him to the hospital. With his parents at his side, he "walked into the hospital, and that was the last time I was able to ambulate on my own" (Sass, 1996, p. 62). None of these young men suspected at the time that these walks would be their last; they all assumed they would recover and walk out of the hospital under their own power.

Increasing paralysis was characteristic of acute poliomyelitis, but so was excruciating pain. Unlike spinal cord injuries where individuals lose both the ability to move and the ability to feel in the body below the injury, polio patients lose the ability to move, but retain the ability to feel. The virus attacks only the motor nerves and not the sensory ones. Almost all accounts of acute polio recall the intense pain associated with the paralysis of the muscles. It was painful to lie in bed, to be covered by a sheet, or to be touched by the nurses. Dorothea Nudelman recalled that "all of it was unspeakable—the stiffness, fever, chills, and agony of being moved, even touched, for a change of bed sheets or night shirt. Total paralysis was like being trapped in a nightmare where you waited to wake up" (Nudelman, 1994, p. 40). Charles Mee remembers a "relentless pain, like the pain of tooth being drilled without novocaine, but all over my body." Mee, like most polio patients, was "not given any painkiller" because "the pain medication might somehow cause additional damage" (Mee, 1999, pp. 17–18). Many of the most effective pain killers work on the central nervous system. With the central nervous system under attack during acute polio, doctors did not want do anything that might increase the rate or extent of paralysis. As a consequence, the severe pain of acute polio had to be borne without any relief.

Older polio patients who remember more of the acute phase of the disease recall entering a kind of netherworld in which they were not quite sure what was real and what was not. The pain, the fever, and the workings of the poliovirus sometimes produced hallucinations and a sense of unreality. For Charles Mee "time slowed to a drift. There were no events outside my own body to orient me to the world's news, family activities, the passing of the day or night—just this endless drift inside myself, with the occasional sound, the opening or closing of a door, the impression of something white and starched going quickly past my bed, the rush of water in the sink, the awareness that it was nighttime in the room" (Mee, 1999, p. 19). When Dorothea Nudelman raised her eyes, she "saw frightening images dancing on the ceiling. I was very hot and thirsty. I woke and slept for what felt like days. I dreamed I was next to a restaurant kitchen, hearing the clatter of dishes and other harsh noises. Then I was on a sailing ship, rocking back and forth unsteadily. Faraway noises pushed at me through a fog, muffled rhythmic pulsing of heavy machinery" (Nudelman, 1994, p. 39). Caught in the grip of acute polio, patients in their hallucinations transformed the ordinary sounds of the hospital into all kinds of fearsome images.

CARING FOR ACUTE POLIO PATIENTS

Doctors and nurses found caring for acute polio patients difficult, especially during severe epidemics when the hospitals were admitting several new patients a day. During the polio epidemics in Minneapolis in 1948 and 1949, Dr. Richard Aldrich likened working on the polio wards to his service in the military during World War II. The doctors and nurses organized themselves into two teams to try to deal with the "steady stream of patients coming in." They tried to divide up the work so they could get some rest, but Aldrich recalled that "it was like being in combat. You have to be on the ball and ready to go all the time. You were tired, exhausted, and frightened at the same time. We didn't want to get polio ourselves" (Seavey, 1998, pp. 114–115). The doctors and nurses were also worried about carrying polio home to their families. During a severe epidemic, "you were essentially on call all the time. It was a total emergency day and night, day after day after day for weeks" (Seavey, 1998, p. 116). Thomas Daniel was a fourth-year medical student when he first worked with polio patients in a Boston hospital. He did what he could to help the patients "through an illness for which there were no curative therapies, no magic bullets, no wonder drugs." He acknowledged that "the care of polio patients was not easy" but also admitted that while physicians "provided medical care," it was the "skilled nurses" who "undertook their work under the difficult circumstances of dealing with paralyzed and frightened patients" (Daniel, 1997, pp. 84, 88).

Juanita Howell was an African American nurse who worked during the polio epidemic in Mississippi in 1946. She recalled that the nurses wore street clothes to and from the polio hospital so as not to alarm others on the bus they rode to and from work. Once they changed into their hospital "scrub-gown," they went on to the polio wards. They tried to help the polio patients as much as possible: "We would wipe their tears, we would wipe drool, we fed them, we brushed their hair, we bathed them, we took care of body elimina-tions, everything. We'd move their fingers, position their hands—some of them were paralyzed and could not move their hands. . . . It was that kind of thing, just kind of common sense, doing what was necessary to make a person feel comfortable. There was no medication. There was no proven anything at that point in time" (Seavey, 1998, pp. 147–148).

There was nothing physicians could do to alter the course of the disease. Physicians and nurses were advised to keep the patients as comfortable as possible. The hospital staff tried to ensure that the polio patients rested, but the pain of polio often made that difficult. By the late 1940s, some hospitals used hot packs of wet wool blankets to try to relieve the muscle pain so common in the acute phase. Polio experts warned against any use of sedatives or pain killers because they could mask the progress of paralysis and doctors needed to be able to determine what parts of the body were becoming paralyzed. This was particularly crucial if the paralysis began to affect the muscles that enabled the patients to breathe.

In addition to caring for their patients, doctors had the difficult task of talking to the parents or the spouse of the polio victim. For Dr. Richard Aldrich, that was "the worst part of the whole thing. . . . Those were some of the most awful experiences I ever had in my life" (Seavey, 1998, p. 115). While physicians like Dr. Aldrich tried to reassure parents that their child would likely recover and that the chances of them dying were small, no doctor could accurately predict at the time of diagnosis how a case of polio would proceed. Patients, parents, and physicians would all have to wait until the disease had run its course before they could begin to assess how much damage and destruction the poliovirus had done.

BULBAR POLIO AND THE INABILITY TO BREATHE

Polio could affect any of the motor nerves in the body. The disease, however, was seldom fatal unless it attacked the nerves that control the muscles used in breathing. When that happened, the patient quickly lost the ability to breathe on her own, and unless assistance was immediately available she died. Until the late 1920s, there was nothing doctors could do to keep patients alive who had lost the ability to breathe independently. In 1928, Philip Drinker, an engineer at the Harvard Medical School, invented the tank respirator, or, as it was more commonly known, the iron lung. Although widely feared by patients and parents, the iron lung saved many lives by assisting polio patients in breathing until they regained the strength to breathe again on their own. Still, the large yellow or green iron lungs and the characteristic "whoosh-whoosh" sound they made while operating remain powerful memories for those who lived through the polio epidemics.

A polio patient's ability to breathe freely could be affected in two ways. In patients with spinal polio, where the poliovirus damaged nerves in the spinal cord, breathing could be impaired if the nerves controlling the muscles that expand and contract the chest were damaged or destroyed. These patients usually benefited from being placed in an iron lung. Patients who had bulbar polio were more seriously impaired. Bulbar polio affected the brain stem and the nerves of the face and head that control swallowing and breathing. The iron lung was not always effective in cases of bulbar polio, and about 60 percent of such patients died even if they were placed in an iron lung. Some individuals had both spinal and bulbar polio, and the mortality rate for these patients was especially high.

The iron lung was a large, human-sized steel tank. At the foot end of the tank was a flexible bellows, often made of leather that could move in and out, thus changing the air pressure in the tank. The head end of the iron lung had a hole in it through which the patient's head stuck out. The patient lay on a cot attached to the head of the tank. The patient was placed on the cot and doctors guided his head through the hole, which was surrounded by a rubber collar to cushion the patient's neck and to provide a tight seal when the iron lung was closed. Once the patient's head was through the hole, the cot with the patient on it would be wheeled into the iron lung and the end would be sealed and latched. The patient's body would be encased in the tank with only the head outside. When the machine was turned on, it moved the bellows at the end of the tank in and out at a rhythm set by the doctor. When the bellows moved out, the air pressure in the lung was reduced and air was drawn into the patient's lungs. When the bellows moved in, the air pressure in the iron lung was increased, forcing the air out of the patient's lungs. Windows and portholes on the sides of the iron lungs gave nurses and physicians access to the patient's body to provide necessary care. A mirror was attached to the iron lung above the patient's head so she could see what was happening behind her.

Because every patient's polio was unique, the onset of respiratory failure differed significantly from patient to patient. Some patients slowly lost the ability to breathe, while others lost respiratory function very quickly. Doctors and nurses carefully monitored the breathing of polio patients so they could be placed in iron lungs if failure occurred. Most polio wards had iron lungs available, and the March of Dimes stood ready to ship additional iron lungs to communities in the midst of a severe epidemic. Many polio survivors recall seeing the empty lungs in hallways awaiting their next occupant and hearing the rhythmic "whoosh-whoosh" of the iron lungs operating somewhere on the hospital floor. Dr Robert Eiben, who worked with polio patients at the contagious disease hospital in Cleveland, Ohio, thought it was "unlikely that there was ever a polio patient who was not fearful of the 'iron lung.'. . . A number of patients acknowledged that they thought going into the tank respirator meant almost certain death, and others equated the machine with a coffin in which they would be buried" (Eiben, 1997, p. 104).

Some placements in the tank respirators went easily. Marilynne Rogers was nine when she contracted polio in Minnesota. On her third day in the hospital, doctors concerned about her breathing told her they were going to put her in a machine to help her breathe. Nurses wheeled her "into this small room, and there was this big machine." She remembers "they opened the respirator; it seemed really huge, and they laid me on the tray with a mattress on it, and then they slid me through the hole at the front of the big roller part. Then they closed up the collar, and told me to really relax. They told me I'd feel much better, and I did. I could breathe more easily" (Sass, 1996, pp. 55–56). Rogers doesn't remember much about the next few weeks, but her medical records reveal that she was in and out of the iron lung. Although her breathing ability recovered sufficiently to allow Rogers to spend time out of the lung, she slept in the iron lung for the rest of her life.

Other placements were much more difficult. Hugh Gallagher's paralysis had begun in his legs. Two days after entering the hospital, polio paralyzed his arms and hands, and he found it increasingly difficult to swallow. Even though the hospital had put him in an oxygen tent, he had increasing difficulty breathing and he kept asking the nurses to check that the oxygen was on. He "lay there, concentrating upon each breath. Each breath became a conscious decision, an exhausting labor, less and less satisfying, ever more tiring." The doctors acted quickly by summoning a specialist to the hospital. He decided to perform an immediate tracheotomy without even taking Gallagher to the operating room. A tracheotomy opens a hole in the trachea below the vocal cords so doctors can insert a silver breathing tube into the trachea. They can then introduce oxygen directly into the lungs. Because Gallagher was too sick for anesthesia, the operation was performed with him fully awake and aware. He watched his throat being cut in the reflection from the doctor's glasses. As soon as the trachea tube was inserted, hospital attendants lifted Gallagher off his mattress and ran with him down the hall to the room housing the iron lung. As he says, "[my] last memory is of being laid out on the pallet and inserted into the tin can of the iron lung," and then he passed out from lack of oxygen. When he regained consciousness, he discovered he was "a prisoner of the iron lung" (Gallagher, 1998, pp. 29–32).

Living in an iron lung was difficult for both the patient and the nurses who provided the necessary care. Hugh Gallagher recalled that his early weeks in the iron lung were hard work: "I and my nurses, for I had two private duty nurses a shift, were very busy. At times, they were frantic. It is surprising how much work is involved in maintaining blood transfusions, glucose intravenous feedings, oxygen supply, catheterization, ice packs, hot packs, the endless adjustments to the body and the equipment—needs that followed one another throughout the day and night" (Gallagher, 1998, p. 34). Nursing such patients required a "highly expert level of professional nursing care" (Dunphy, 2001, p. 14). Jim Marugg's nurses "watched and tended" his body "as if it were an expensive and complicated machine. . . . Its air intake controlled by the faithful respirator. Its calculated amount of nourishment injected into it without the effort of chewing and swallowing. Its waste removed by enemas and catheters and throat pumps" (Marugg, 1954, p. 54).

Nurses had to work on the patients through the open portholes, which reduced the effectiveness of the iron lung, or slide the patient out of the lung for the few minutes he could breathe on his own. Encased in the lung, patients like Gallagher could do nothing for themselves. They had to be fed. If they itched, they had to be scratched. Men had to be shaved, and both men and women had to have their hair combed. Their tears needed to be wiped and their noses blown. Urinals and bedpans had to be inserted into the lung and taken away. Their most important task was "the maintenance of a patient airway." If the throat muscles were paralyzed, as they often were in bulbar polio, nurses frequently had to suction out the nasal and throat secretions so that the patient would not choke on them. Nurses found it "physically exhausting in actual physical energy expended to care for the patient and it is a mental strain trying to imbue him with confidence and a hopeful outlook" (Dunphy, 2001, pp. 20–21). One of the most terrifying moments on polio wards occurred when the power in the hospital went off because of a lightening strike and the iron lungs stopped. The respirators could be pumped by hand, but it was hard work, and when the power went out "maintenance people, gardeners, sweepers, anybody who was available, came to help do that" (Seavey, 1998, p. 151). Most people could only operate an iron lung manually for a few minutes before they handed the machine off to the next volunteer. Thankfully, most iron lung patients could breathe a few minutes out of the lung. In addition, most hospitals had emergency generators so that the power was quickly restored and the machine could resume its rhythmic pumping once again.

While a few individuals used an iron lung for three or four decades, most polio patients were weaned from the iron lung within a few weeks or months of their acute attack. Nurses opened the lung and slid the patient out for a minute or perhaps two or three. Sometimes nurses also performed part of their care routine outside of the lung, which was easier to do.

The patient tried very hard to breathe on his own, but it wasn't easy, especially at the beginning. Kenneth Kingery, an Air Force officer stricken on his last day in the service, recalled that when nurses opened the iron lung he "made a horrifying discovery": he had "to *work* to breathe." He dreaded the opening of the tank because, as he said, "I'd have to strain my every fibre for a breath of air. And there was always a helpless terror—wondering whether they'd close the tank in time." Each day, the nurses lengthened the time Kingery spent outside the lung so that his chest muscles could begin to recover their strength and he could once again breathe independently. These episodes outside the lung were also supposed to build the patient's confidence in his recovery, but Kingery disagreed: "Whatever confidence I gained from these fish-out-of-water torture trials came *after* each tank opening. Never before" (Kingery, 1966, pp. 49, 51). Hugh Gallagher felt that his nurses were expecting too much of him when they put him on a strict iron lung weaning schedule: "I had learned to take a breath, perhaps two. Now, she said, the time would be doubled from 30 seconds to a minute. After I had breathed a minute, the time would be upped to two minutes; and then she said, each day's time would be doubled." He recalled that "it seemed impossible. It was like telling a goldfish it could walk." In spite of his protests, "the therapist's plan went like clockwork. The driving schedule, just one more painful and frightening event in the day, went on inexorably." Still, he had to admit that "the muscles that were responsible for breathing were able to meet the challenge. I was actually breathing on my own" (Gallagher, 1998, pp. 51–52). Some five weeks after being put in the tank, Gallagher was moved to a separate bed. That first day he stayed on the bed only an hour before being moved back to the iron lung, but before long he was out of the machine altogether.

Not all iron lung patients were successfully weaned of their dependence on the machine. Some died in the weeks after being slid into the tanks. Perhaps the poliovirus had done too much damage, and the machine could not compensate. Or perhaps secretions clogged the airway and were not suctioned in time. Others died of pneumonia or other respiratory infections. Nurses and other attendants tried to prevent other polio patients from being aware of the death of a ward mate, but there were signs that all of them recognized. A familiar "whoosh-whoosh" was suddenly stilled, and an iron lung was wheeled into the hall. In some hospitals, when an iron lung patient died, the "death signal was the passing of a nurse down the row of tanks, turning each mirror so the patients couldn't watch while a body was wheeled out in a now silent machine" (Black, 1996, p. 64).

INITIAL RECOVERY FROM ACUTE POLIO

While some patients with respiratory failure died during the acute stage of polio, most survived. The length of the acute illness varied from patient to

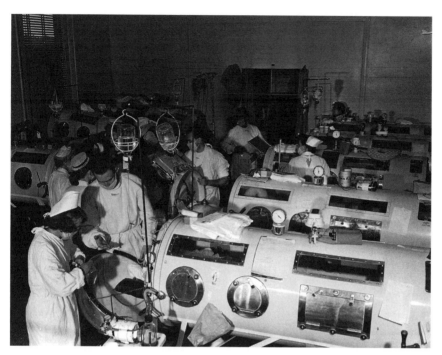

Polio patients in an iron lung or respirator ward at Haynes Memorial Hospital in Boston, Massachusetts, during the 1955 polio epidemic. (March of Dimes)

patient, but generally lasted ten days to two weeks. The acute phase ended after the poliovirus had ceased to destroy nerves and the patient's fever had subsided. Doctors typically waited forty-eight hours after the patient's temperature had returned to normal before deciding that the acute illness had run its course. These patients, especially in severe cases, were still very sick. Some had run a high fever for days. Some had lost consciousness or had hallucinations at the height of the illness. Most had experienced significant muscle pain as the muscles were weakened and paralyzed. Many still had significant paralysis. These patients were also still contagious as they continued to shed the poliovirus in their bowel movements for several weeks following the end of the acute illness.

The end of the acute illness usually meant that the polio patient was moved from the isolation facility to a convalescent ward or room in another part of the hospital. This freed up a bed in the isolation ward, an important consideration in an epidemic with new cases arriving daily. Convalescent patients also needed somewhat less care than acute patients, although those with substantial paralysis still required careful attention from the nursing staff since they could do so little for themselves. Doctors and patients could begin to assess the extent of the damage, although at this stage of the illness it was still impossible for physicians to predict accurately how much of the paralysis was permanent and how much could be lessened or eliminated by rehabilitation.

Once polio patients were out of isolation, visits from parents and spouses resumed, although visiting hours were often quite restrictive in these years. Visiting hours were often only an hour or two, and in some hospitals, visitors were allowed on only two or three days of the week. These visits were eagerly awaited by patients, who missed their families and the support they offered. At visiting time, all the patients listened intently for one distinct sound. As Charles Mee later recalled, "Everyone I know has one memory vivid above all others: the sound of their mother's high-heeled shoes in the hallway—utterly distinct from the shoes of anyone else's mother—when she came to visit" (Mee, 1999, p. 26).

Polio patients rightly regarded the move to convalescent wards as a step toward returning home. However, few understood how long it would be and how much work it would take before they would be able to leave the hospital and return to their families. Patients with mild cases of polio might return home after a few weeks or perhaps a month of rehabilitation. But those whose paralysis was more extensive could spend months, sometimes years, in rehabilitation before they had achieved the maximum possible recovery. Still, most welcomed the move as it meant they were slowly getting better.

8

Convalescent Polio and Rehabilitation

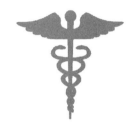

Many polio patients at the time of their initial illness expected to be hospitalized for at most a week or two and then return home fully recovered. They were often disappointed because the recovery from polio and the rehabilitation of muscles damaged by the disease were usually long and difficult. Still, polio patients regarded moving out of the acute ward and isolation as a milestone. They were feeling better. The pain and fever had receded. Visitors were now allowed and no longer had to wear masks and hospital gowns when they came. Most polio patients were moved to hospital rehabilitation wards that housed between four and twenty patients, often arranged by sex and age so that patients were quickly introduced to a new set of friends who had been through a similar ordeal and had survived. These ward companions helped maintain morale during both the difficult exercises and the long hours spent on the ward between visits to the hospital's rehabilitation facility.

Both the physicians and the patients found polio rehabilitation long and challenging. Doctors usually made an initial assessment of the damage done by the disease at the time patients were transferred to rehabilitation. However, their initial assessments were tentative at best. Polio-damaged muscles could take up to two years to recover maximum possible function. Rehabilitation was designed to strengthen those muscles only weakened by polio. Rehabilitation also involved finding ways to compensate for those muscles permanently paralyzed by the disease. This compensation might mean training other unaffected muscles to substitute for the paralyzed ones. It might mean surgery to transplant working muscles and tendons or to correct deformities of the spine and other bones caused by uneven muscle strength. When neither exercise nor surgery provided adequate compensation for paralyzed muscles, polio patients were taught to use assistive devices such as braces, crutches, and wheelchairs. For patients in iron lungs, rehabilitation meant increased efforts to lessen their dependence on the iron lung and to increase the amount of time they could breathe on their own without any mechanical assistance. The goal of this rehabilitative regime was to get polio patients to a point where they could go home and function in the family and at school or work.

In addition to the physical challenges of polio rehabilitation, these patients also had to deal with psychological trauma. Only a few weeks before, they had been healthy children or young adults. Now, they had survived a serious illness, but parts of their bodies were still paralyzed. Perhaps they could not walk, feed themselves, or dress themselves. Perhaps their breathing was impaired and they needed the assistance of an iron lung. They needed to come to terms with being disabled and with uncertain prospects for a full recovery. The rehabilitation period was often long and hard, and many polio patients endured long separations from their families while trying to regain the use of polio-affected muscles. And when doctors decided that the formal period of rehabilitation had ended, many polio survivors were still left with significant disabilities they would have to live with. Unfortunately, in the period of the polio epidemics, there were few psychiatrists, psychologists, or other mental health professionals available to help polio patients adjust to their disabilities. Most had to face the future with only the help and support of family and friends.

REHABILITATION FACILITIES

Polio rehabilitation occurred in a wide variety of settings and institutions. Some hospitals that treated acute polio patients also had rehabilitation wards so that when the time came to move to rehabilitation, the patients simply had to move down the hall. Other polio patients were transferred to state- and community-supported rehabilitation facilities that had been established many years before to provide care for individuals with physical disabilities. During the years of the polio epidemics in the mid-twentieth century, polio patients made up a majority of the individuals in these hospitals. Examples of these institutions were the state-supported Gillette Children's Hospital in Minneapolis, Minnesota, and the New York Reconstruction Hospital north of New York City.

There were also county institutions such as Rancho Los Amigos in Los Angeles County, California. Private facilities also existed, such as the Sister Kenny Institute in Minneapolis and the hospitals for crippled children run by the Shriners in a number of states. The most famous polio rehabilitation facility, of course, was the Georgia Warm Springs Foundation established in 1928 by Franklin Roosevelt. Some rehabilitation institutions, such as Rancho Los Amigos and Warm Springs, were regarded as state-of-the-art facilities. Others, however, especially some of the state-run facilities, were bleak, inhospitable institutions that provided substandard care. African Americans often had a difficult time finding a good rehabilitation facility, especially in the south, where hospitals were segregated and state support for black institutions was substantially less than that for hospitals serving white patients.

Where patients underwent rehabilitation depended on the severity of their paralysis, the income of the family, the place where they lived, and their race. Warm Springs was the most famous polio rehabilitation facility, and it was one of the best. However, it was small, with a patient population of around one hundred. Well funded by the Georgia Warm Springs Foundation and the March of Dimes, Warm Springs by the early 1940s was both well staffed with trained professionals and well equipped. It was also permeated with the spirit of Franklin Roosevelt, who continued to return to his institution until his death in 1945. Roosevelt always insisted that Warm Springs retain something of its heritage as a resort and that the staff address the psychological and emotional dimensions of rehabilitation as well as the physical ones. Hugh Gallagher caught something of the character of Warm Springs when he recalled his transfer from a hospital in Washington, D.C. to Georgia: "The difference between life as a patient in the old hospital and rehabilitation at the beautiful resort, deep in the Georgia pines, was as great as the difference between Kansas and Oz" (Gallagher, 1998, p. 71). Warm Springs was probably the only rehabilitation facility that could plausibly be described as a resort, but relatively few polio patients were ever treated there, and all of them were white.

THE ETHIC OF POLIO REHABILITATION

The polio epidemics occurred at a time in the United States when the Protestant work ethic was still strong and physical therapy following polio drew upon the cultural influence of that ethic to motivate polio patients. The sociologist Fred Davis identified the importance of the Protestant work ethic for polio patients: "The physiotherapy regime, which in its very design faithfully captures the essence of the Protestant ideology of achievement in our culture—namely, slow, patient, and regularly applied effort in pursuit of a

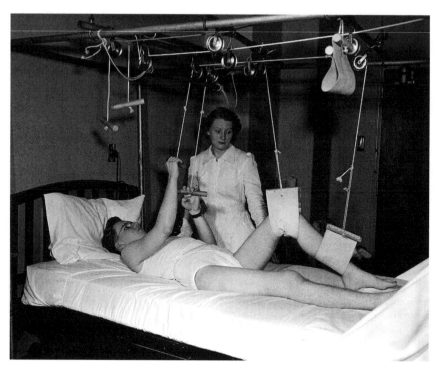

A young man in 1950 exercising in bed using pulleys and weights as part of his rehabilitation from polio. (March of Dimes)

long-range goal—has built into it, as it were, its own prophecy of success" (Davis, 1991, p. 71). This ethic worked so well in part because children and adolescents had already been exposed to these values at home and in school. The Protestant work ethic resonated with the ethic of polio rehabilitation because each day's achievement in the gym or the swimming pool was small. Over time, however, these small improvements added up to recovery.

Anne Finger, who had polio when she was three, felt the influence of this polio ethic during her rehabilitation. She recalls that the therapy gym was full of "plaques and posters with inspirational sayings: 'The only place where success comes before hard work is in the dictionary.' A drawing of the tortoise crossing the finish line before the hare. 'Slow and steady wins every time.' A drawing of a ladder, on whose bottom rung were the words 'I can't do it,' followed by 'I might try, but just once.' 'I am trying to do it, but it hurts,' and finally ending with 'I did it'" (Finger, 2006, p. 118).

Edward LeComte was a Columbia University professor when he contracted polio on a trip to France. But, like Anne Finger, he felt the influence of the polio ethic: "Every day in the gymnasium I was expected to do something terribly dangerous—such as going four steps further—that I hadn't done before. They called it progress: that was the iron rule." Le Comte, however, also resented the up beat message from the posters and the therapists: "I disliked intensely the moralizings that were flung at us. 'Mary did it—you can do it.' Didn't it depend on how much either of us the virus had eaten? But, as is likely to happen with incessant propaganda, some of it stuck. Maybe there were indeed borderline cases where, 'whether you ever walk again *is up to you!*'" (Le Comte, 1957, pp. 96–97). However they felt about the "incessant propaganda," most polio patients were unwilling to risk failing in their rehabilitation, so they spent day after day at their exercises, slowly trying to regain the use of their muscles.

STRETCHING AND HOT PACKS

As polio patients moved from acute care to convalescent and rehabilitative care, doctors faced the challenge of trying to prevent the characteristic deformities caused by the disease at this time. Most of the muscles of the body operate in opposing pairs that enable us, for example, to bend at the elbow or knee. The poliovirus often weakened or paralyzed one of a pair of muscles. Meeting no resistance from the paralyzed muscle, the stronger, undamaged muscle would contract. As the acute phase of the illness ended, therapists tried to stretch contracted muscles, particularly in the arms and legs, so as to prevent permanent deformity. This often painful process could take weeks before full range of motion was achieved. Before the 1940s, polio patients were often put in splints or casts once the muscles had been stretched to prevent a recurrence. However, after the arrival of the Australian nurse Sister Elizabeth Kenny, many doctors and therapists switched to using hot wool packs to loosen contracted muscles, to aid in stretching, and to prevent permanent deformities. Virtually every polio survivor from the 1940s and 1950s remembers weeks of therapy with the hot packs until their muscles had sufficiently stretched.

During the early twentieth century, doctors had relied on splints and casts to prevent muscle contractures and permanent deformity. Once the arm or leg had been stretched to achieve normal extension, the limb would be put in a splint or cast to maintain this extended position. The patient might spend several weeks or even months in these splints and casts until the physician determined that further contractures were unlikely. Long-term splinting and casting, however, brought its own set of problems. Healthy muscles that are not used for a long time, such as when they are in a cast, begin to weaken and atrophy. Polio survivors who spent long periods in these casts emerged with muscles paralyzed from polio and with other muscles atrophied from lack of use. Dr. John Paul described the 1930s as an "era when early and prolonged splinting of paralyzed limbs was carried to excess" (Paul, 1971, p. 338). By the early 1940s, some physicians had begun to adopt hot packs and massage as alternatives to casting to prevent deformities. This change was hastened by the arrival in the United States in 1940 of Sister Kenny, who was a powerful advocate for hot packs.

Elizabeth Kenny was an Australian nurse who developed her method of treating polio patients while working in isolated rural Australia. She became known as Sister Kenny, following the way nurses were typically given titles in British hospitals. Kenny had discovered that hot packs of wet wool applied to polio patients with contracted muscles lessened the pain and loosened the muscle so that the therapist could stretch it more easily. She also developed her own theory of polio. She believed that it was a muscle disease, not a nerve disease, and that the muscles had become alienated from the brain. As a result, the muscles had spasms that created the deformities of polio. The hot packs relaxed the muscles so that the therapists could begin to stretch them and move them through their range of motion. If a patient was unable to move the limb herself, the therapist would move it for her to re- educate the limb by reconnecting it to signals from the brain. Physicians never accepted Kenny's theory about polio or her notion of alienation, but they discovered that the hot wool packs were effective in reducing pain and loosening the muscles so they could be more easily moved by the therapist and eventually by the patient.

Kenny was a powerful advocate for her beliefs, first in Australia and after 1940 in the United States. She met significant opposition from physicians in both countries who discounted her theories and initially rejected her methods of hot packs and passive exercise. The mostly male doctors of the period were reluctant to acknowledge that a female nurse could develop an effective treatment for polio. Kenny, however, found supporters in the medical community, especially in Minneapolis, where she eventually established the Sister Kenny Institute to provide care using her treatments and to train therapists in her methods. Even though doctors rejected her theories of what caused the deformities of polio, by the late 1940s, most accepted that Kenny's methods of treating patients with hot packs during both the acute and rehabilitative phases of the disease lessened the pain of polio and made it easier for therapists to prevent deformities.

The Kenny treatment was memorable for every one who endured it. Charles Mee described it as "such a bizarre, disgusting procedure that no one who had polio in those days has forgotten what seemed like a punishment for having gotten sick. The blankets itched, of course, and were either so hot to begin with that they scorched and burned—mere warmth was never considered sufficient—or else they got cold and clammy in short order" (Mee, 1999, pp. 64–65). For Brenda Serotte, "the badge of a courageous child was taking the Sister Kenny treatment as hot as they gave it without weeping or whimpering. I'd compete with myself every day to do better than the day before and not make a sound. But even the boys cried out, it was so painful." Serotte remembers that "everyone in the beds suddenly stopped talking mid-afternoon each day, when the aluminum carts rattled toward us." The carts were plugged in to heat the water producing, as Serotte says, the "steaming-hot woolen cloths. Then just at that temperature, they'd be placed on our paralyzed legs." The wet wool was so hot that the nurses fished the cloths out of the carts with wooden tongs so they would not get burned. The wool was then usually run through a wringer to get rid of excess water before being placed on the patient. Sometimes, nurses covered the wool with plastic sheeting to help retain the heat. Serotte recalls that when the wool cooled off, "then you'd be shivering—but not for long. In a half hour or so the nurse returned, and some freshly boiled flannels were applied" (Serotte, 2006, p. 108). Polio struck most often in the summer, but most hospitals in the 1940s and 1950s had no air conditioning. That meant that the hot packs were endured in hot, steamy wards where the temperature might already be in the eighties. Although the nurses tried to be careful, sometimes the wool was just too hot and the patients were burned. Dorothea Nudelman tried "to believe I wouldn't get burned, but, when it happened, I sobbed out loud, wore myself out with it. The shock was as bad as the pain. I knew it could happen again" (Nudelman, 1994, p. 60).

The stretching of contracted muscles was often as painful as the hot packs, especially at the beginning. Robert Hall remembers watching a ward mate being stretched by the physical therapist. The therapist was "forcefully stretching Putzie's hamstrings by pushing the foot down, maybe even tearing them." Hall watched the "beads of perspiration spring up on Putzie's forehead as he turned his head in pain. . . . Then he screamed. . . . I believe all 250 patients in our hospital heard Putzie's scream" (Hall, 1990, p. 66). Not all stretching was so brutal. Charles Mee's therapist, Mrs. Jones, was "far, far gentler—spreading out the pain in smaller increments over some weeks." She began and ended every session massaging his muscles. She started with his hands and feet and then lifted his arms and legs off the bed. Mrs. Jones "worked gently, diligently, patiently to repair my body as much as she could and to dissolve my sense of hopelessness" (Mee, 1999, p. 68).

In addition to the hot packs and stretching, some hospitals used tubs of hot water, hydrotherapy, to loosen muscles and to use the buoyancy of the water to help patients move their affected limbs. Mee recalls being taken down to the therapy room where male attendants lifted him on to "a cloth stretcher, which was lowered by a winch into a whirlpool bath the size and shape of an angel in the snow" (Mee, 1999, p. 68). Warm Springs, of course, was famous for its use of hydrotherapy. The warm spring water bubbling out of the hillside into the pools had initially attracted Franklin Roosevelt to the site. Even when he returned to Warm Springs as governor of New York and as president, Roosevelt exercised in the warm pools and played games with the polio patients then in attendance.

Once the hot packs, stretching, massage, and hydrotherapy had sufficiently loosened the patients' muscles, they could begin physical therapy to rebuild strength in those muscles that were only weakened by polio. Physical therapy might begin in the patient's bed on the ward to get him to a point where he could go to the gym for more extensive exercises. For Charles Mee, as for so many other polio patients, progress was slow. After a week of hot packs, he had become "flexible enough to have my head propped up on pillows so that I could see around my whole room." Eventually he moved the fingers on both hands, and then lifted his left arm off the bed by himself. Finally, a month after leaving isolation and after two weeks of work with his therapist, Mee turned over in bed by himself. After another two weeks, he sat in a wheelchair for the first time and moved about his room and into the hallway. In the physical therapy gym he lifted weights to build strength in his arms and shoulders so that he could pull himself to a standing position some two months after entering rehabilitation (Mee, 1999, pp. 69–70).

LEARNING TO WALK AGAIN

Regaining the ability to walk was a key goal for both patients and therapists. As Brenda Serotte observed, "the blessed walked out of the hospital on their own power; the cursed were pushed out" (Serotte, 2006, p. 73). Polio could paralyze any muscle in the body, but it seemed to have a particular fondness for the leg muscles. Learning to walk again was the goal of every polio survivor whose legs were affected, but it was often a long, painful process that did not always succeed. Serotte's therapist told her that she would "soon be walking on [her] own without any braces whatever," which is what Serotte wanted to hear. But before she could learn to walk, she had to learn to fall so as not to hurt herself, falls being inevitable: "We were taught that there was an art to falling, so we fell, on purpose, time after time. If we balked, they'd push us back down again, harder." Serotte also had to figure out a way to get up off the floor by herself, a skill she finally mastered. The therapists pushed

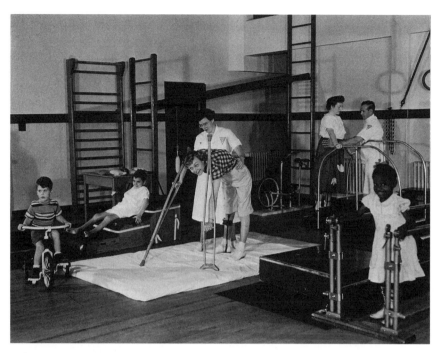

Polio patients exercising their muscles and learning to walk again in a rehabilitation facility in 1952. (March of Dimes)

Serotte and the other polio patients as far as they could, and sometimes beyond: "Fight! Fight! Fight! was, would always be, the polio theme song. There was no such thing as feeling sorry for yourself, crying, or saying 'it hurts.' Unless you wanted to be a 'helpless cripple,' synonymous with 'hateful devil,' you fought, you fell, you climbed, you stretched, you kept working." When she took her first steps, it felt like "walking on top of a shaky bed." After four months in bed, she "had lost completely not only the ability to automatically move my legs but also the memory of what real walking felt like. I yearned for it. We all did, and we'd all strive for just that, to walk like we used to, as if polio had not occurred" (Serotte, 2006, pp. 166–169).

Boys as well as girls struggled to regain the ability to walk. Like many polio patients, Charles Mee's goal "was to be a real person who could walk. Walking was the whole deal." But it was not easy. He recalled that "whenever you did see someone begin to walk again—so awkward, fragile, and dangerous an enterprise—it seemed a miracle" (Mee, 1999, p. 95). He took his first awkward and fragile step some three months after he had been carried into the isolation ward. And then three weeks later, after much practice and many falls, he walked the length of the hospital corridor outside the therapy room for the first time.

Not everybody whose leg muscles had been affected could learn to walk again; sometimes too many muscles were permanently paralyzed. Jan Little ultimately decided that walking was impossible. She, like most polio patients, had tried for many weeks to develop the muscles and techniques to walk again, but it was hopeless. As she recalled, her therapists would "prop me up on braces that reached to my waist, re-enforced by a corset that reached to my armpits and we would practice walking." Most of the time, however, Little "imitated a tree;" she would "sway back and forth a few frantic moments, then crash to the ground, maintaining a straight position," all the while falling. Nothing she and the therapist tried worked, and Little and her family ultimately decided that she would need to rely on a wheelchair for mobility (Little, 1996, pp. 11–12).

While these polio patients were trying to learn to walk again, other patients whose polio had affected other muscles were going through similar exercises in an effort to regain function. They might be trying to regain arm or hand strength so they could feed and dress themselves or write or type. They might be exercising the muscles of the torso and abdomen so they could sit unaided or in the attempt to prevent scoliosis, a curvature of the spine so common among polio survivors. And in respiratory centers across the United States, patients in iron lungs were trying to learn to breathe again unaided by mechanical respiration.

WEANING FROM IRON LUNGS

Weaning patients from iron lungs began as soon as the patient's fever broke, but it could take weeks, sometimes months, for patients to regain sufficient muscle strength to breathe for significant lengths of time without assistance. Doctors wanted to lessen the patient's dependence on the respirator as quickly as possible for both safety and convenience. The longer a patient could breathe on her own outside the lung, the safer she was in case of a power outage. It was also easier for the nurses to care for patients outside the iron lung, rather than having to work through open portholes. Patients who had grown dependent on the iron lung to breathe for them were not so sure they wanted to leave the safety of the respirator. As Hugh Gallagher put it, "I was, once established on the iron lung routine, reasonably comfortable and not anxious to alter my circumstances" (Gallagher, 1998, p. 51).

Therapists used several techniques to wean patients from iron lungs. As we saw earlier, nurses began almost immediately sliding patients out of the lung

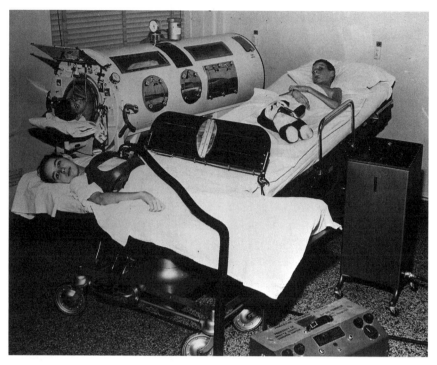

Polio patients whose respiratory muscles were paralyzed depended on machines to breathe for them or to help them breathe. The most seriously affected required an iron lung (top). As their breathing recovered, they might be moved to a rocking bed (middle) or a chest respirator (bottom). (March of Dimes)

for brief periods of time to test their breathing ability and to care for them. As the patient's breathing capacity returned, the therapists lengthened the time out of the lung from a few minutes, to half an hour, to several hours, to a whole day. Even when they could spend a day outside the iron lung, many patients continued for some time to sleep in the respirator. Returning to the iron lung at night gave their tired chest muscles time to recover from the exertions of the day. Therapists also taught some respirator patients the difficult technique of glossopharyngeal breathing, or, as the polio patients called it, "frog breathing." Frog breathing used the tongue and neck muscles to force air into the lungs in imitation of the way frogs were supposed to breathe. This was difficult to learn and required a conscious effort to maintain, but patients whose chest muscles were paralyzed and who learned to frog breathe had a margin of safety if the iron lung lost power. At his best, Louis Sternburg could frog breathe for fourteen hours straight, but, as he said, "it took tremendous energy and effort" and he was "exhausted at the end of each session" (Sternburg, 1986, p. 65).

As their muscle strength returned, some of these patients were moved to rocking beds. These beds were like large teeter-totters on which the patients lay. As the head of the bed went up, gravity pulled the internal organs down and the patient breathed in. As the foot of the bed went up, gravity pushed the internal organs up on the diaphragm and pushed the air out of the lungs. Rocking beds provided less respiratory support than iron lungs, but they helped many patients in the transition to breathing on their own. It was easier to care for patients on rocking beds, and the beds gave patients a wider field of view. In spite of the incessant rocking, patients soon adjusted. For Louis Sternburg, moving to a rocking bed meant he was making progress in his goal of leaving the iron lung. He worried that it wouldn't provide sufficient support and that he would get seasick, but he was relieved to discover that it made possible a "more natural type of breathing, less forceful than the iron lung," and he quickly concluded that it was "a triumph, Another way to breathe, another choice" (Sternburg, 1986, p. 39).

Some hospitals also used chest respirators, which were small respirators that fit around the chest and abdomen. These were powered by electricity or batteries and allowed patients to sit up, to be in a wheelchair, and to have some mobility. Some patients were allowed to go on home visits with chest respirators before they were ready to be permanently discharged. At Rancho Los Amigos in Los Angeles, married polio patients who went on home visits in a chest respirator usually asked for an Emerson rather than a Huxley machine. When the hospital staff inquired about this choice, they discovered that because of the way the machines fit on the body, "the patients could have sexual relations with an Emerson. They couldn't in a Huxley" (Seavey, 1998, p. 142).

Because caring for patients in iron lungs was so difficult, the National Foundation in the late 1940s and early 1950s established fifteen respirator centers around the country and moved many of the patients living in iron lungs to these centers. These centers provided trained physicians, nurses, and therapists and a higher level of care than could be provided in many community hospitals. By 1953, these centers had accepted over 300 patients, many of whom had been dependent on iron lungs for months. The improved care at these centers meant that "within a year, the several centers were able to discharge 80% of the patients home; almost half of them were completely weaned from the machines, and the remainder were able to use smaller aids (like the chest devices), some or all of the time" (Rothman, 1997, p. 63). The success of these respiratory centers helped give rise to the creation of intensive care units in hospitals in the 1950s and 1960s.

While many iron lung patients were able to leave the respirators after a few weeks or months, others lived dependent on the machine for years. Mark O'Brien was six in 1955 when polio left him paralyzed from the neck down and dependent on an iron lung. He graduated from the University of California at Berkeley, became a published poet and writer, was the subject of an Oscar-winning documentary, and wrote his autobiography before dying in 1999. In 2008, there were perhaps twenty individuals still dependent on the iron lung to breathe for them, but today many other polio survivors rely on other forms of respiratory assistance such as ventilators to support their breathing.

Most people who contracted polio did not die from the disease, but patients whose breathing was affected were at the greatest risk. Before the development of the iron lung in the late 1920s, patients who lost the ability to breathe invariably died because medicine had no effective means to help them. Even with the iron lung, some polio patients died because their paralysis was so severe. This was especially the case with patients who had both bulbar polio that affected their neck and throat muscles and spinal polio that affected their chest muscles. Some patients, like Virginia Black, recovered sufficiently to be sent home with a rocking bed and chest respirator, only to die soon after. Doctors didn't always know why such patients died when others lived many years in the respirators. Iron lung patients often had serious medical issues like kidney stones and respiratory illnesses such as pneumonia, but those who died shortly after leaving rehabilitation also appeared "to lack the initiative, drive, imagination and support systems to achieve what the more successful patients had" (Black, 1996, p. 246).

SURGERY

Physicians preferred to use physical therapy to rehabilitate bodies ravaged by polio. But not all deformities could be alleviated through hot packs and exercise. Although some patients had surgery soon after leaving the acute hospital, most polio patients did not enter the operating room until two or more years after their illness struck. It could take up to two years for a polio patient to regain maximum function through physical therapy, and doctors generally preferred to wait to see how much progress could be made with therapy before considering surgery. Surgeons also preferred to wait until their younger patients had achieved most of their growth before operating. Many polio patients spent their teen years in and out of the hospital for a series of operations. Orthopedic surgeons performed a number of different kinds of operations. Among the most common were tendon and muscle transplants in the hands, arms, legs, and feet. These operations moved a functioning tendon or muscle to a new position to compensate for tendons and muscles paralyzed by polio. These surgeries allowed patients to grasp things with their hands, to write, to use their arms more effectively, and to walk more easily and safely. Spinal fusions were probably the most dramatic of the polio surgeries. Here, physicians used body casts to straighten the curved spines of patients and then fused the straightened spine with bone or metal rods to maintain a properly aligned spine against the unequal pull of paralyzed and healthy muscles.

Because these surgeries occurred some years after the initial illness and the completion of physical rehabilitation, polio survivors often found them particularly difficult to endure. They had returned home and to school, attempting to resume their interrupted lives. They were not eager to return to the hospital and to endure the pain associated with surgery. But return they did. As Dorothea Nudelman put it, "The hospital was like summer camp for polios. Surgeries were planned. You booked a spot in advance." Still, it was hard: "The worse part, though, was going into the hospital feeling healthy and pretty and then experiencing pain and bodily violation in a way that was totally debilitating. It was like losing it all over again, only this time I wasn't a little kid anymore" (Nudelman, 1994, pp. 134–135).

Spinal fusions were perhaps the most difficult and protracted of the surgical procedures performed on polio patients. I remember going into the hospital in the summer of 1960 when I was ten. I was first taken to the casting room, where my entire torso was encased in a plaster cast. Attached to the cast were two metal bars with a screw. Once the cast dried and I was back in the hospital bed, the doctor began to straighten my spine. Every day for several weeks he would come into my room and turn the screw slightly, each time straightening my spine a little more. At this point I experienced no pain because each day's adjustment was so small. After my spine was straight, the surgeon cut a hole in the back of the cast and, using bone taken from my left leg, fused the vertebrae of the spine in the straight position. After a week or so to recover from the surgery, I was sent home in my body cast to recover. My parents set up a hospital bed in the living room, and I spent the next several months flat on my back while the spine healed. But at least I was home with my family, and a visiting teacher came weekly to keep me up with my fifth grade class.

As teenagers, many polio patients made their own decisions regarding possible surgery, and sometimes they chose not to have the operation. For example, Charles Mee's physician proposed fusing the bones in his left leg to stabilize it and make walking easier. However, the fusion would make sitting normally impossible. After talking with his parents, Mee decided against the surgery (Mee, 1999, pp. 175–176). Many of the choices these patients made involved improving one function through the surgery, walking for example, but making another useful function, such as sitting normally, almost impossible. In weighing the options, polio patients often decided to accept less function in one area to maintain function in another activity. Also, by the time they were in their late teens, many of these patients had had several surgeries. They were unwilling to put their lives on hold again for the marginal benefit surgery would provide. They decided to make do with what function they had and get on with living.

LIFE ON THE POLIO WARDS

Most polio patients who underwent polio rehabilitation in a hospital spent long hours on the polio wards that housed from four to twenty patients. Hospital stays were longer in the 1940s and 1950s, and it was typical for polio patients to spend anywhere from several weeks to several months or even a year or more in a rehabilitation hospital. These long hospital stays meant that a community of polio patients often developed on the wards because while patients were always coming and going, you would be surrounded by the same group of patients for most of your stay. These wards were typically segregated by age and sex so that there were wards for older boys and men and another for younger boys and separate wards for older girls and women and for younger girls. New polio patients on the ward found it easy to make friends since everyone had been through similar experiences.

Communities developed on these wards because of the shared experience of polio, because the patients spent many hours together between therapy sessions, and because by the time polio patients reached rehabilitation they were no longer sick. Parts of their bodies might be paralyzed and not work terribly well or at all, but the illness had passed. To be sure, there were the physical pains of rehabilitation and the psychological pain of being separated from family and friends, but their ability to play, think, laugh, and have a good time was not impaired. Where these polio communities developed, they did much to ease the burdens of polio rehabilitation.

When Larry Alexander moved to a six-bed men's ward at the Sister Kenny Institute in Jersey City, New Jersey, he experienced "a comforting feeling in the presence of other men, in the constant talk, the arguments, and the horseplay" (Alexander, 1954, pp. 84–85). At Warm Springs, Hugh Gallagher found that he "could have fun again" (Gallagher, 1998, p. 74). Not all moves to the rehabilitation wards went so easily. When doctors moved the nineteen-year-old Lorenzo Milam to rehabilitation, he was still recovering from the acute illness and not really ready to face the ward community. He found himself overwhelmed "in a football-field-length medical ward with noise from 6:30 a.m. to 9:30 p.m. non-stop. Noise: babbling, calling out, yelling, whistling, stomping, running, singing, crying" (Milam, 1984, pp. 18–19). Like Gallagher, he, too, found things more to his liking at Warm Springs.

Some younger children quickly found themselves part of the ward community. Arvid Schwartz was twelve when polio struck. When he was moved to a rehabilitation hospital, he worried about how he would fit in. There were "all those strange faces, all young boys approximately my age, ten to fifteen. And I thought, 'I don't know anybody in here.'" Soon, however, another patient, Dave Jenkins, introduced himself and helped Schwartz get used to life on the ward (Seavey, 1998, p. 256).

Newcomers to the rehabilitation ward learned an important lesson by discovering that others had survived acute polio and were, in many cases, farther along in their recovery from the disease. When fifteen-year-old Irving Zola was transferred to the all-male polio ward where he would ultimately spend six months in rehabilitation, his "spirits rose almost immediately." He was "warmly welcomed as the 'new polio,'" and he was relieved to see others in similar situations. Even more important to Zola was "seeing some patients actually move about," as it gave him hope for his own recovery (Zola, 1983, p. 9).

Patients on the polio wards not only welcomed the new patients, but also helped one another in a variety of ways. Most polio hospitals lacked sufficient nurses and attendants to provide all the care for their paralyzed patients. As a result, polio patients who had regained some mobility or had the use of their arms assisted other patients whose recovery was just beginning. They might scratch someone's itch, turn pages in a book, or light a cigarette. Polio patients also taught one another techniques for transferring from a bed to a wheelchair and other useful skills. Physical therapists provided some instruction in these skills, but it was often easier for a patient to master these necessary skills after seeing how someone with a similar impairment managed the feat.

Polio patients also helped one another deal with the psychological impact of paralysis and the hard work of rehabilitation. Irving Zola recalled that one of the benefits of the polio ward was that he was "surrounded by fellow patients in varying degrees of a struggle, each cheering the others on" (Zola, 1983, p. 15). While this encouragement helped many polio patients endure the weeks and months of rehabilitation, others found it more oppressive. Charles Mee, for example, found that "this culture made me feel, as a boy, that I needed to keep my chin up, reassure my parents about how well I was doing, never be sad, look to the future, be optimistic, perform a can-do persona even if I felt no connection to it" (Mee, 1999, p. 93). Even though he rejected the ideology of the ward, Mee persisted with his exercises.

Because so many polio patients were children and teenagers, and because many spent months in rehabilitation hospitals, most of the larger institutions made some provisions for them to continue their education. Some set up class-rooms and brought in teachers, while in others, patients were tutored individu-ally. These classes were designed to keep the polio patients up on their education so that when they left the hospital they could return to their grade and their familiar classmates.

Exercises, hydrotherapy, and school took time out of each weekday, but polio patients spent many unoccupied hours on the ward. They tried to enter-tain each other in a variety of ways. Most wards had radios, and listening to favorite shows occupied many hours. Television was in its infancy during the polio epidemic, and it was only in the mid-1950s that televisions began to appear on polio wards. Many of the larger hospitals provided a regular movie night when the patients would be moved to the hospital auditorium or gym to watch the film.

Patients also read, played games, and used their imaginations to fill the many long hours. They enjoyed playing pranks on one another and on the nurses and hospital attendants. Many polio patients discovered that if they stuck the end of the paper covering the plastic straws in soft butter, they could then blow very hard and the paper would fly to the ceiling and stick. Some ward ceilings were covered with a whole forest of hanging paper. Other patients made sling-shots with rubber bands and used paper spitballs as ammunition.

As polio patients became more mobile in wheelchairs and on crutches, they began to explore the hospital corridors. Mobility also meant that one could visit the wards of the opposite sex. Both boys and girls discovered that wheel-chairs were good for racing, at least until someone ran into a nurse or a hospi-tal cart and everyone was grounded for a few days. Increased mobility also enabled some patients to get outside for the first time in months. Many hospi-tals had patios or other areas where patients could gather on nice days and enjoy the sun.

While polio patients generally appreciated the efforts of the nurses, thera-pists, and attendants, almost every hospital had one or two members of the staff whom the patients resented. Perhaps they had a gruff tone, or they interpreted the hospital regulations very strictly and punished patients for minor infrac-tions. It wasn't unusual for the ward to conspire to take their revenge on staff they felt treated them badly. Robert Hall remembered that he and his friends carried out a campaign against "Old Crotchety": "It was war forever, undeclared war, against her. Whenever we could we made life miserable for her. I really believed all of this added to our determination to get well. Her presence stimu-lated a constant, added adrenalin production" (Hall, 1990, p. 86).

Warm Springs had perhaps the most developed social life for its patients. In part, this was a legacy of its founding by Franklin Roosevelt, who wanted it to retain the atmosphere of the resort it had once been even as it became a leading center of polio rehabilitation. Hugh Gallagher recalled that Warm Springs "provided an opportunity to meet people, undertake joint activities, make friends, date, and fall in love. The whole range of normal social activities went on at Warm Springs, much the way it does in the rest of the world. New patients were welcomed into the group. Their handicap did not isolate them from the norm; it *was* the norm" (Gallagher, 1998, p. 81). No other polio rehabilitation facility could have been described as resort-like, but something similar happened at most larger polio rehabilitation hospitals. As they rebuilt their bodies in the exercise gyms, polio patients restored their ability to live and work in the community outside the hospital through their social life in the ward community.

Most polio wards were welcoming places, especially following the harrowing experience of acute polio. But no matter how many new friends these polio patients made, they still missed their families and friends from home. The loneliness that many polio patients experienced during rehabilitation was made worse by the very restrictive visiting policies of most rehabilitation hospitals in the 1940s and 1950s. A few institutions were very liberal in their visiting hours, but most places limited visiting to a few hours on one or two days of the week. Other places were even more restrictive. The Shrine hospital in San Francisco, for example, permitted the parents of patients to visit only on Sundays for a half an hour, and parents were not allowed to come together. Other hospitals took away patients' visiting privileges if they had misbehaved or if parents fell behind on paying the bills (Wilson, 2005, p. 125). The limited visiting hours were made worse because parents and spouses were not always able to take advantage of the hours that were available. Polio rehabilitation often took place in hospitals that were many miles away from the patients' families. Distance, work, and bad weather often made it impossible for family to visit weekly. Phone contact was also limited as not all wards had phones for public use and long-distance calls were expensive. Phones were generally used only in emergencies. By the time polio patients were in rehabilitation, they were no longer contagious. There was no medical reason for such limited visiting hours, except for the convenience of the hospital.

Holidays spent in the hospital were particularly difficult. Many institutions tried to make it possible for patients to spend a few days at home over Christmas or Thanksgiving, but it wasn't possible in every case. For those who remained in the hospital over the holidays, the staff tried to get the ward in the spirit of the season. Wards were usually decorated for Christmas, and many had a tree. Families brought presents, and often service organizations provided additional presents and seasonal entertainment, such as a visit from Santa Claus, for the hospital-bound patients. Still, it wasn't like being at home.

After weeks and months of exercises, tears, loneliness, and fun with new friends, rehabilitation came to an end. It was time to go home. Doctors and therapists usually made the decisions to discharge patients when they had achieved all that physical therapy and surgery could do. Patients had rebuilt strength in the muscles that remained and had learned to compensate for those permanently paralyzed. If necessary, they had learned how to walk on braces and crutches, and how to fall without hurting themselves. Others had begun to adapt to life in a wheelchair. Respirator patients had learned to breathe again on their own for at least part of the day, but many went home with rocking beds or chest respirators to assist breathing, particularly while sleeping. A few even went home with their iron lungs. While some were disappointed that they were unable to walk out of the hospital on their own, all were glad to be leaving for home.

Leaving the rehabilitation hospital did not mean the end of recovery. Polio patients could recover muscle function up to two years after the initial illness. Many patients and their families were instructed how to perform exercises on their own that would continue to build strong muscles. Others went to outpatient therapy several times a week or found swimming pools where they could exercise in the buoyant water. Others found themselves returning to the hospital in coming years for surgeries to correct what physical therapy and exercise could not. Whether someone walked out without assistance, was wheeled out in a chair, or went home with a list of prescribed exercises, all were happy to have this phase of their recovery behind them.

9

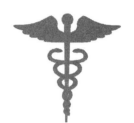

The Search for a Polio Vaccine

Jonas Salk's development of the polio vaccine was one of the most celebrated events of twentieth-century medicine. Salk's picture was on the cover of *TIME* magazine, and newspapers across the country hailed him as a modern hero who had vanquished a dreaded disease. While Salk's achievement represented a modern medical triumph, his success was the product of long-sustained and well-financed effort on the part of many scientists and physicians to first understand the poliovirus and how it worked in the body and then to develop a successful vaccine against it. The National Foundation for Infantile Paralysis (NFIP) played a key role in this effort. Money raised by the March of Dimes funded almost all of the scientific and medical research that lay behind the polio vaccines. Although the March of Dimes did no medical research itself, its grants made the research possible and gave it considerable influence over the direction of polio research. From its very beginning, the goal of the NFIP had been to develop a successful polio vaccine as soon as possible. But it would take more time, money, and research than anyone imagined in 1938 when the National Foundation was created.

THE NATIONAL FOUNDATION FOR INFANTILE PARALYSIS AND THE CAMPAIGN AGAINST POLIO

The National Foundation for Infantile Paralysis was not a scientific agency. As we have seen, Franklin Roosevelt and Basil O'Connor created the foundation in 1938 to raise funds to support the facility at Warm Springs, Georgia, as well as to support research on the poliovirus and provide assistance to victims of the disease in their home communities. O'Connor realized that the National Foundation had to avoid a disaster such as the failed 1935 vaccine trials of Dr. Brodie and Dr. Kolmer. Since he was a lawyer and not a scientist, O'Connor decided to get the best medical advice he could to establish a program of financial aid to polio researchers. He needed a superb virologist who knew the field, who would give him straightforward advice, and who had credibility with men and women conducting research on polio. He asked Dr. Thomas Rivers, director of the Rockefeller Institute Hospital in New York, to head the scientific research committee. Rivers was a prominent virologist and careful scientist who lent his authority to this new organization dedicated to eliminating polio.

The Committee on Scientific Research of the NFIP came into being on July 6, 1938. It was composed of five physicians, including three virologists and the medical writer Paul de Kruif, who had served on a similar committee for the President's Birthday Ball Commission. The committee elected Dr. Rivers as chairman, a position he would hold for seventeen years. They quickly set about regularizing the process of applying for funding. The committee surveyed the field of polio researchers to establish what was already known about the disease and what needed to be learned to create a successful and safe vaccine. From the responses, Rivers compiled a list of problems and questions that needed attention. The Committee on Scientific Research then listed the problems in the order of their importance. The Committee ranked discovering the "pathology of poliomyelitis in human beings" first and learning the "portal of entry and exit of the virus" second. Other key problems were uncovering the "mode of transmission of virus from man to man" at number five, and "transmission of virus along the nerves" at six. "Production of a good vaccine" was last on Rivers' eleven-point list (Benison, 1967, p. 232). As this list of problems about polio suggests, scientists still lacked a full understanding of the disease. There was still some uncertainty about how the poliovirus worked in the human body. The scientists were not sure whether the nose or the mouth was the entry point for the virus, although learning that would enable them to pinpoint how the virus left the body to infect others. In 1938, no scientist expected to see a safe and effective polio vaccine developed any time soon.

The Committee on Scientific Research funded both individual scholars and university laboratories focused on polio research. For example, Dr. Albert Sabin received a grant to study how polio entered the body. The polio research laboratories at Yale University, the University of Michigan, and Johns Hopkins University also received funding from the committee. The Committee gave scientists at Yale and Michigan grants to explore the epidemiology of polio, how it operated in the community, and how it spread from human to human. The polio laboratory at Johns Hopkins focused its study on the pathology of polio, in particular how it infected the central nervous system, where it did its damage (Oshinsky, 2005, p. 60). The arrival of the funding from the National Foundation proved to be a mixed blessing. On the one hand, the generous grants from the March of Dimes enabled scientists to expand their research into polio and to up grade their laboratories and staff at a time when there was almost no government funding of medical research. As Dr. John Paul, one of the scientists on the Yale Poliomyelitis Unit, recalled, the NFIP appeared to polio researchers as a "fairy godmother of quite mammoth proportions" (Paul, 1971, p. 311). On the other hand, as Paul also acknowledged, since the National Foundation provided the money, they had considerable say in what kinds of polio research were undertaken.

Dr. Rivers was one of the key figures in the NFIP's scientific grant program, but he was not the only one. Harry Weaver, the National Foundation's director of research from 1946 to 1953, played a central role leading the NFIP's grant program and thus shaped polio research in the late 1940s and early 1950s. Before joining the National Foundation, Weaver had been professor of anatomy at Wayne State University in Detroit where he had conducted research on polio and nutrition. Dr. Rivers credits Weaver with being "bold" and an important "catalyst" for polio research (Bension, 1967, p. 405). As David Oshinsky observed, Weaver focused on "removing the obstacles that had been stalling polio vaccine progress for years" (Oshinksy, 2005, p. 113). Weaver introduced two important innovations into the grant-giving process. First, the National Foundation grants were structured to cover some of the indirect costs of the universities where polio research was being done. Indirect costs are those things not directly related to the scientific research such as maintenance, gas and electric costs, and payment of staff such as janitors and others needed to keep the buildings running. Weaver developed a formula to add a certain percentage to each grant to cover these indirect costs. Weaver's second innovation instituted multi-year grants so that the scientists would not have to reapply every year for funding. These multi-year grants reduced paperwork and allowed the researchers to plan long-term research confident that it would be funded (Oshinsky, 2005, pp. 113–114).

The appointments of Rivers to oversee the scientific quality of the funded research and Weaver to direct the research program gave the National Foundation the key personnel to disburse its funds most effectively. While Basil O'Connor never lost sight of his ultimate goal of creating an effective and safe vaccine, he relied on his scientific advisors who recommended first funding basic virological research before tackling the difficult task of creating a good vaccine. Much polio research was deferred during World War II since many of the scientists and physicians were called into the military, where they conducted research to protect soldiers and sailors from a variety of bacterial and viral diseases. When the war ended in 1945, the National Foundation prepared to launch a new effort to eliminate the threat of polio.

BASIC RESEARCH ON THE POLIOVIRUS

Because there were so many unanswered questions about polio, as Dr. Rivers' eleven-point list of research topics suggests, many of the early March of Dimes grants went to scientists exploring the basic biology and pathology of the poliovirus. These basic grants focused on three areas: first, determining how many different strains or varieties of polio existed in the wild; second, conducting clinical research to determine how polio entered and exited the human body and how it spread in communities; and third, determining how to grow the poliovirus in the large quantities required to produce a vaccine.

Scientists needed to determine how many strains of polio existed in nature if they were ever going to develop a vaccine. Exposure to one strain of a virus conveys immunity to future infections from that strain of the virus, but not from other strains of the same virus. If there were a small number of poliovirus strains, developing a vaccine would be simpler because scientists would have to create only a limited number variations on the vaccine to protect against all the possible strains. If, however, there were many independent strains of poliovirus, then the challenge of making a virus became much greater because, again, the vaccine would have to protect against each of these many strains.

In 1931, two Australian researchers, Frank M. Burnet and Janet Macnamara, discovered that there were at least two distinct strains of poliovirus. They demonstrated conclusively that exposure to the first strain did not convey immunity to the second. This was an important finding since it alerted scientists to the possibility of multiple strains of polio. However, in the wake of the Australians' discovery, scientists made no immediate and concerted effort to find out whether additional strains existed. Six years later, the polio research group at Yale confirmed Burnet's and Macnamara's discovery of two distinct strains of poliovirus (Paul, 1971, pp. 227, 231). But this still left unanswered the question of how many additional strains might exist.

After World War II ended, the National Foundation for Infantile Paralysis put a high priority on settling the question of the number of poliovirus strains. At a 1946 conference sponsored by the National Foundation, scientists and physicians began to plan how best to determine the number of poliovirus strains. They agreed that a cooperative program held the most promise of success. In July 1948, another NFIP conference drew up plans for the research and appointed a committee to oversee these plans' implementation. Beginning with some 250 samples of poliovirus drawn from a variety of sources, the Committee on Typing of Strains selected 100 strains for study, 86 of which came from the United States and the rest from elsewhere. Several laboratories were chosen to perform the work, including those of David Bodian at Johns Hopkins and Jonas Salk at the University of Pittsburgh. Typing poliovirus strains was dull and repetitive work but absolutely vital to the success of any vaccine. Ultimately, an additional ninety-six strains were added to the original group for a total of 196 samples tested.

After several years of hard work in these laboratories, the scientists concluded that there were only three strains of poliovirus. As mentioned in Chapter 5, Type I made up 82.1 percent of the samples, Type II constituted 10. 2 percent, and Type III was the rarest at 7.7 percent. The Committee on Typing had overcome many obstacles to come up with these results. National Foundation funds were used to expand laboratories, pay staff, and purchase the many monkeys needed to test the various strains of the virus. Dr. Jonas Salk and his laboratory at the University of Pittsburgh were key players in the typing program. Dr. John Paul regarded the typing project as a "major triumph for the NFIP to have engineered this cooperative endeavor among a highly individualistic group of research workers" (Paul, 1971, p. 235). As he noted, "It represented the first interuniversity venture in poliomyelitis research in which eight members of a committee, who directed four laboratories, pooled their brains and resources in the interest of a common problem." Equally important, this venture provided a model for future National Foundation funding efforts against polio. The typing program, Dr. Paul wrote, "provided a vision of future accomplishments to be implemented through its advisory committees and facilities. A major strategy for leading the fight against infantile paralysis to its ultimate conquest had begun, with Dr. Rivers as a commanding figure" (Paul, 1971, p. 239).

The second line of attack supported by the March of Dimes' money explored the clinical pathology of poliomyelitis. That is, it addressed the question of how the poliovirus operated in the human body from the time of infection until the virus was released to infect another person. Although Swedish researchers had done some work in this area early in the twentieth century, their research had been largely ignored in the intervening decades. The work of Dr. Simon Flexner and others had established the prevailing belief that polio entered the body through the nose and proceeded to the spinal cord along nasal nerves. Flexner and others had been able to experimentally infect monkeys using this route and assumed that the origin of infection in humans was the same. There was some scattered evidence from Swedish researchers and others that the mouth and throat were the port of entry for the polio virus in humans, but the kind of systematic study that could dislodge the orthodox view was not carried out until the 1930s.

During the 1937 polio epidemic in New Haven, Connecticut, the Yale Poliomyelitis Unit demonstrated that the poliovirus could be isolated from throat specimens and from stool samples, or fecal material. In one family of three children in which the oldest child had a case of paralytic polio and the youngest an apparent mild and non-paralytic case, researchers found poliovirus in three stool samples from the youngest child, the last of which was tested more than three weeks after the onset of his illness. Dr. John Paul, who participated in this study, wrote that it was easier to find poliovirus in stool samples than in throat samples because the amount of virus present was considerably larger and the virus remained in the stool longer than in the throat. As he observed, "The results implied that the virus had not been merely swallowed but that multiplication in the alimentary tract continued for at least several weeks" (Paul, 1971, pp. 280–282). The discoveries of the Yale group would be confirmed by other studies in subsequent years. This evidence strongly suggested that the mouth was the point of entry for the poliovirus, that it multiplied in the intestinal tract, and that it was shed in fecal material to infect new victims. This was important information both for advising individuals how to avoid infection and for developing a vaccine.

As more scientists began to study stool samples during polio epidemic, it became apparent that individuals who showed no paralytic symptoms were significant carriers of the disease. In addition, researchers discovered that "inapparent carriers were more common in infants and pre-school children than in those of school age, and infinitely less common in adults." These discoveries gave support to a growing consensus that "a great deal of poliovirus infection lay completely below the surface" and that very young children might provide a "huge reservoir of virus" during any polio epidemic (Paul, 1971, p. 286). It was becoming much more evident that the individuals paralyzed in any polio epidemic were only a small percentage of the individuals infected.

A number of authorities had blamed the spread of polio in the great 1916 epidemic in New York on flies that carried the disease from the sick to contaminate the food of healthy individuals. The theory of fly transmission of polio remained credible into the 1940s. Then, during that decade, a number of experiments demonstrated that reducing the fly population did little to reduce or stop a polio epidemic. The Yale Poliomyelitis Unit participated in an experiment during the 1945 epidemic in Rockford, Illinois, in which large amounts of the insecticide DDT were sprayed on the city from the air and by hand. As Dr. Paul observed, this "resulted in a temporary reduction of flies, but ... it had no effect on the progress of the poliomyelitis epidemic." A similar experiment in Texas in 1948 produced the same negative result, and by the early 1950s, spraying against flies during polio epidemics was largely abandoned (Paul, 1971, p. 297).

In the 1930s, scientists developed techniques to test blood serum for antibodies to the poliovirus. Blood serum is the yellowish liquid that remains when the blood solids, such as red blood cells, are removed. The blood serum carries the antibodies to the viruses that we have been exposed to, and the ability to detect and measure antibodies in blood sera gave researchers a new tool to test for the poliovirus. This tool enabled scientists to conduct serological surveys to test the blood serum of a large number of individuals for antibodies to the poliovirus. This gave them a much more precise tool to determine the spread of the virus. When doctors began conducting these serological tests in the 1930s, they demonstrated that "most infants are born with short-lived, passive antibodies, derived from their mothers." After infants lost this protection, many began to "acquire active antibodies and immunity through inapparent infection." The evidence suggested that at age "fifteen between 80 and 100 percent of children are antibody positive and presumably immune" to polio (Paul, 1971, p. 358). This meant that when the poliovirus was in regular circulation, as it was in areas without modern sanitation, almost all adolescents and adults were immune to polio because they had had an inapparent case while very young. In countries such as the United States, where modern sanitation interrupted the constant circulation of the poliovirus, epidemics occurred because not every child was naturally immunized by maternal antibodies.

One of the other unanswered questions about the poliovirus had to do with where it resided in the body between the time it entered through the mouth and the time it entered the central nervous system to do its damage. Doctors who treated polio patients and who conducted clinical research on those patients had suspected that there was first a "generalized infection," and that at some point the virus appeared in the blood of an infected person. But no one had been able to isolate poliovirus in the blood from a polio patient or from an experimental monkey. Part of the problem was in using monkeys for the research. Most experimental monkeys were infected by introducing the virus into the nerves of the nose, where it had a direct nerve pathway to the spinal cord. This experimental method of infection bypassed the bloodstream entirely. But as growing evidence revealed, this is not how humans are infected with poliovirus. Humans are infected through the mouth by way of contaminated food or dirty hands. By the late 1940s, researchers had induced polio by feeding the poliovirus to cynomolgus monkeys, one of the monkeys typically used for scientific research, and to chimpanzees. Dr. Dorothy Horstmann and her Yale colleagues demonstrated that when the blood of these experimental animals was tested during the incubation period, between the time of infection and when the animal began to show signs of the disease, they could detect the virus in the blood, a condition known as viremia. This suggested that the same might apply to humans. During the 1952 polio epidemic, Dr. Horstmann and her colleagues collected blood samples from families in which there was a case of paralytic polio. They hoped to collect blood from other family members who might be in the incubation state or in the initial stages of the disease. When they tested this blood, they were able "to isolate virus from the blood during the incubation period with some regularity in the human infection" (Paul, 1971, p. 389). The discovery of viremia in humans was important because "it meant that small amounts of virus which invaded the blood could probably be overcome by relatively small amounts of circulating antibody, and by this means could be blocked from gaining access to the central nervous system." This also had important implications for developing a vaccine. As John Paul put it, "At one fell swoop the problem of immunizing man had been rendered easier than was expected" (Paul, 1971, p. 389).

Scientists developing a vaccine still faced a major hurdle, how to grow sufficient poliovirus to make millions of doses. Unlike bacteria, which will grow on a variety of nutrients, viruses will multiply only in cell tissue. This makes the cultivation of viruses much more difficult. The poliovirus proved particularly difficult to grow, but unless some means were found, a vaccine would be impossible to create. The earliest attempts to grow poliovirus succeeded with a strain of the virus adapted to monkeys. This strain, however, had become so adapted to nerve tissue that it would only grow there, which made it impracticable for vaccine production.

The obstacles to growing poliovirus were finally overcome in the laboratory of Dr. John Enders at the Children's Hospital in Boston. Enders worked with two younger colleagues, Dr. Thomas Weller and Dr. Frederick Robbins. The three scientists used tissue cells that were finely cut and suspended in a nutrient fluid that was changed every four days. The laboratory had been attempting to grow the viruses that produced measles and chicken pox. One day in

1948, Enders suggested that they try some of the poliovirus stored in a freezer. As Dr. Robbins remembered, "Much to our amazement the virus grew, not only in brain tissue but in skin, muscle, kidney, and intestine." They originally used human kidney tissue taken from infants undergoing a medical procedure requiring the removal of one kidney. Later the researchers discovered that monkey kidneys worked equally well. Dr. Robbins recalled that "although it appeared that the virus was really growing in the cultures; it was some months before we could convince ourselves that this was true" (Robbins, 1997, pp. 126–127). In addition to discovering that they could grow poliovirus in non-nerve tissue, Enders, Robbins, and Weller also discovered that, as the poliovirus multiplied, it caused a particular change in the cells of the tissue culture. This made it possible to detect the presence of poliovirus in tissue cultures using only a high-powered light microscope. The discoveries of Enders's laboratory were important because they made it possible to grow large amounts of poliovirus and because it made it possible to test for the presence of poliovirus in a Petri dish rather than having to inject monkeys with possibly infected material to see if they would develop polio (Paul, 1971, p. 374). Testing in a Petri dish was both faster and far less expensive. In 1954, Enders, Robbins, and Weller received the Nobel Prize in Medicine for their discoveries.

By the early 1950s, many of the mysteries of the poliovirus that in 1935 had prevented the development of a safe and effective vaccine had been solved. Scientists knew there were only three strains of polio, not dozens. Clinical research had revealed how the poliovirus operated in the body, including the important fact that it could be found in the bloodstream shortly after infection. Polio was also revealed to be an intestinal disease that was taken in the mouth and shed in the stool of infected individuals. Finally, Enders, Robbins, and Weller had demonstrated that it was possible to grow poliovirus in non-nervous and readily available tissues. Thus, by the early 1950s the stage was set for another attempt to create a successful polio vaccine.

JONAS SALK AND THE DEVELOPMENT OF HIS POLIO VACCINE

Basil O'Connor's goal had always been to support the development of a vaccine as soon as it was possible. He understood and accepted the need to know more about the poliovirus and how it operated in the body before creation of a successful vaccine was feasible. O'Connor, however, continually pushed his scientific and medical advisors to approve grants that moved the development of a vaccine forward as quickly as possible. By the late 1940s, there were several scientists and laboratories working on vaccine development. Dr. Jonas Salk at the University of Pittsburgh would ultimately produce the first successful polio vaccine, but his triumph was by no means assured as the decade of the 1940s came to a close.

Medical scientists were working on two different types of vaccine: a killed-virus vaccine and a weakened, or attenuated, live-virus vaccine. A killed-virus vaccine uses a chemical, such as formalin, to kill the virus in such a way that it cannot cause the disease but retains sufficient viral characteristics to produce an antibody response in the body. The antibodies produced by the body's immune system provide protection when the body is later infected by the poliovirus, thus preventing the disease. Doctors administered this vaccine with an injection, or shot. A weakened, or attenuated, live-virus vaccine uses various tissue culture methods to weaken the virus sufficiently so it will not cause a case of paralytic polio. Again, the body, in response to the administration of the vaccine, develops antibodies to the poliovirus, thus protecting the individual from future infection. The live poliovirus vaccine is administered through the mouth. When a doctor administers the live poliovirus vaccine, he is giving the patient a very weak polio infection. Because it is given by mouth, the live-virus vaccine mimics a case of polio but is too weak to do damage. It is impossible to get polio from a vaccine in which the virus has been properly killed. With an attenuated live-virus vaccine, a very small number of cases of polio may appear in individuals with compromised immune systems. There might be one case of polio for every 1 million vaccinations. Each vaccine has its advantages and disadvantages, and in the late 1940s and 1950s, scientists were working on developing both types.

Isabel Morgan at the Johns Hopkins University was one of the medical scientists working on research that could have led to a polio vaccine. Johns Hopkins was one of the leading laboratories for polio research, and by the late 1940s, Morgan was developing a killed-virus vaccine. She used formalin, which was the chemical formaldehyde suspended in a solution, to kill the virus before injecting the vaccine into monkeys. When she later attempted to give the monkeys a case of polio, the antibodies produced in response to the vaccine protected them. She was the first researcher to use formalin to inactivate the poliovirus. However, in 1949, Morgan married and gave up polio research to live and work in New York with her husband (Oshinsky, 2005, pp. 130–131).

Dr. Hilary Koprowski was also developing a polio vaccine in the late 1940s. Koprowski worked for Lederle Laboratories, a major pharmaceutical manufacturer. Koprowski developed a live-virus vaccine that Lederle hoped to be able to market. In the late 1940s he tested a live-virus vaccine on nine chimpanzees. He then fed the chimpanzees strong doses of the same strain of poliovirus. None of the chimpanzees developed polio, which suggested that the vaccine worked. He also tested his vaccine on himself and a lab assistant, with no apparent ill effects. In 1950, Koprowski tested his live-virus polio vaccine on children housed in a nearby state institution for children with epilepsy and other developmental disabilities. Koprowski conducted these tests in secret, and it is not entirely clear what kind of permission he had to experiment on the nineteen children who received the experimental vaccine. Fortunately, none of the children developed polio, and all of the children who were not already immune developed antibodies. When Koprowski reported on his experiment at a meeting sponsored by the National Foundation, he was severely criticized by the other scientists in attendance for rushing human testing and risking an epidemic. Koprowski would continue to work on his vaccine for the next decade (Oshinsky, 2005, pp. 134–136).

Jonas Salk's initial involvement with the March of Dimes came through his participation in the typing program that determined that there were only three different types of poliovirus. Salk and his laboratory did a great deal of the work to test the many samples of poliovirus. At the same time, his laboratory was also doing some preliminary work on a polio vaccine. By 1950, his laboratory had already conducted some experiments with monkeys involving both a killed-virus vaccine and a live-virus one. His laboratory was also experimenting with adjuvants, which were added to the vaccines to make them work more effectively, and with different means of killing the virus such as with formalin or ultraviolet light. Salk also began to explore with the March of Dimes the possibility of conducting human trials in the near future (Oshinsky, 2005, pp. 150–151).

As the typing program came to an end, Salk and his laboratory received a large grant from the National Foundation for Infantile Paralysis. He used the money to expand his lab and to hire new personnel with the goal of finding a way to produce poliovirus in the large quantities needed for vaccine production. Enders, Weller, and Robbins had developed the key methodology of using tissue culture to grow the vaccine, but they had not gone on to develop techniques that would produce the massive quantities of poliovirus needed for a vaccine that could be given to every child in the United States. Salk hired two younger scientists, the microbiologist Julius Younger and the zoologist Elsie Ward, to work on the problem. After trying unsuccessfully to grow poliovirus on tissue cultures derived from monkey testes, they succeeded using cultures of prepared monkey kidneys. Younger also used an established technique to separate the individual kidney cells to provide a greater surface area on which the poliovirus could grow. They discovered that a cell nutrient, Medium 199, developed at Connaught Laboratories in Toronto, Canada, worked well with the monkey kidney cells. To produce the large quantities of poliovirus, monkey kidney cells were infected with the virus. The trays of cells were placed in a rocking incubator to ensure that all the cells were bathed in the nutrient. The scientists periodically changed the nutrient and eventually collected the liquid in large bottles. The lab workers then ran the liquid through very fine filters to eliminate everything in the liquid except the polio-virus (Oshinsky, 2005, pp. 154–155).

Once Salk's lab had developed a successful technique of growing large quantities of poliovirus, they had to decide which particular strains of the virus would be used to develop a vaccine. What they needed, as one observer noted, was a variety "powerful enough to cause immunity and yet docile enough to do no harm" (Oshinsky, 2005, p. 155). Salk was so confidant that his methods of inactivating the poliovirus were effective that, for each of the three types of poliovirus, he chose a particularly virulent and dangerous strain to be the basis for the polio vaccine. As David Oshinsky has written, there was an "art" to inactivating poliovirus. The formaldehyde had to be mixed in just the right ra-tio, the mix had to be kept cold with ice, and it had to be thoroughly mixed so that the mixture reached every particle of virus to inactivate it. Too little formaldehyde or not enough mixing might leave active virus particles capable of causing polio. Too much formaldehyde and the virus particles would not be able to generate an antibody response from the body's immune system. After each batch had gone through this process, samples were tested in monkeys to see if they were capable of developing a proper level of antibody or of trans-mitting the polio. If even one monkey became sick, the entire batch of vac-cine was discarded. Salk claimed that making "polio vaccine was 'one of the simplest medical preparations to manufacture,'" but each stage of the process had to be conducted precisely for the vaccine to be both safe and effective (Oshinsky, 2005, pp. 155–156). Creating a procedure to manufacture large quantities of the vaccine and testing it successfully in monkeys were only the first steps to developing a vaccine for humans.

TESTING THE SALK VACCINE

Salk's next task was to gain support for testing his vaccine, especially from the March of Dimes, which funded his research. In 1951, Harry Weaver, the director of research for the NFIP, created an Immunization Committee to pro-vide advice regarding progress toward a polio vaccine. The twelve-member committee included most of the prominent researchers working on a vaccine, including both Jonas Salk and Albert Sabin. Other members included John Enders, Thomas Rivers, and Thomas Francis. The members of the committee had very different views on the feasibility of a live-virus vaccine versus a killed-virus vaccine and on the wisdom of human trials of an experimental vaccine. In December 1951, Salk presented the results of his successful killed-virus vaccine experiments on monkeys. The next logical step was testing in humans. Although the committee made no recommendations regarding human testing of Salk's vaccine, it was clear from the discussions that most members of the committee believed that an attenuated live-virus vaccine held the best chance for immunization against polio. Many members felt additional research was necessary before human trials were attempted. The lack of a specific recommendation, however, gave Salk and Weaver some room to proceed cautiously and in a limited way with human testing (Oshinsky, 2005, p. 157).

Salk prepared to go ahead with limited human trials at two institutions near Pittsburgh that housed children with a variety of medical problems. The D. T. Watson Home for Crippled Children cared for children with physical disabilities, most of whom had had polio. The Polk School for the Retarded and Feeble-Minded was a state institution for children with intellectual and developmental disabilities. Salk and the NFIP faced the problem of securing consent to the experiment since the subjects of the test were minors. Salk got the consent of many of the parents at the Watson Home, but that proved more difficult at the Polk School, where many parents had little contact with their children after placing them in the institution. Since the Polk School had experienced a recent polio epidemic, the risk of testing the vaccine seemed relatively small. The superintendent of the Polk School sought permission from the State of Pennsylvania to allow Salk's test. The state authorities allowed Salk's experiment to proceed so long as he obtained parental consent where it was possible to do so. Salk began his experiment in June 1952, when he tested the blood of children at the Watson Home who were recovering from polio. Once he determined which type of polio a child had by the antibodies in the blood, he then injected him or her with the vaccine for that type. A child who had Type I polio would be injected with vaccine against Type I poliovirus. Salk's goal was to learn whether his vaccine would safely increase the level of antibodies in the blood, thus providing enhanced protection against polio. He then tested the blood over several months to determine how long this enhanced protection lasted (Oshinsky, 2005, pp. 157–159). Salk tested all three types of polio vaccine on the Watson home volunteers. His first volunteer was sixteen-year-old Bill Kirkpatrick, whose legs had been paralyzed a year earlier by the disease. After giving children the vaccine, Salk carefully monitored their health over the next several months. It was an anxious time for Salk. As he recalled, "When you inoculate children with a polio vaccine you don't sleep well for two or three months" (Oshinsky, 2005, p. 160). The results of the experiment were all positive. None of the children developed polio, and the antibody levels in their bloodstream rose.

The risks were much greater when Salk began inoculating the children at the Polk School. While some of the children had polio antibodies in their blood, indicating they had once been infected and were now immune to that strain of polio, others had no antibodies and thus no immunity. Those with no immunity were at risk of getting polio if Salk's techniques had not inactivated all the poliovirus in the vaccine. According to David Oshinsky, "The Polk findings were even more impressive. The vaccine proved safe. It stimulated a high antibody response to all three types of poliovirus that persisted for months. Salk was ecstatic. 'It was the thrill of my life.' he recalled" (Oshinsky, 2005, p. 160).

In January 1953, Basil O'Connor presided over a meeting of the Committee on Immunization of the NFIP that met in Hershey, Pennsylvania. At the meeting, Salk presented the results of his experimental vaccination of 161 children at the two institutions. Salk's achievement impressed some members of the committee, but the group was deeply divided over how to proceed from this point. Albert Sabin and others remained convinced that a live-virus vaccine was superior to Salk's killed-virus vaccine, but no one, including Sabin, was close to testing a live-virus vaccine. Many of the scientists in the room cautioned Salk and the NFIP to proceed slowly. They felt there were still too many unanswered questions regarding safety and effectiveness to proceed to a large-scale field trial. A few participants urged Salk to conduct a larger field trial, but they were a distinct minority. Dr. John Enders articulated the general view of the committee when he suggested that Salk conduct "more experimentation along the same lines that he is doing so admirably at the moment, and not enter into a large experiment which will inevitably be connected with a lot of publicity and may jeopardize the entire program." Salk seemed to agree, and did not push for approval of a quick field trial (Benison, 1967, p. 496).

Shortly after the meeting adjourned, Dr. Thomas Rivers, chairman of the NFIP's Committee on Scientific Research, met with Harry Weaver, the NFIP director of research, to discuss the advantages and disadvantages of a field trial of the Salk vaccine. Weaver then prepared a document for Basil O'Connor that outlined the issues facing the National Foundation in early 1953. Weaver acknowledged that "the practice of medicine is based on calculated risk," as no decision is ever completely risk free. The ideal, he thought, was "to follow the course that provides the greatest benefit with the least risk of incurring any untoward effects." Not all the possible questions about the safety and efficacy of the Salk vaccine had been answered, and additional research would undoubtedly provide some of those answers. Weaver then posed the dilemma: "If such research is carried out, a very considerable amount of time will elapse before a poliomyelitis vaccine is made available for widespread use; with the

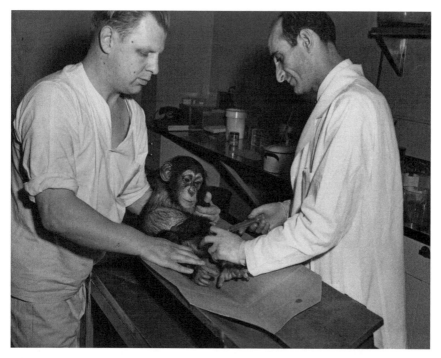

Laboratory technicians in 1952 vaccinate a chimpanzee against polio as part of the research on polio vaccines. (March of Dimes)

result that, in the interim, large numbers of human beings will develop polio-myelitis who might have been prevented from doing so had the vaccine been made available at an earlier date." Weaver believed that the time had come to consider non-scientific, "sociological" factors in deciding whether to proceed with a field trial (Benison, 1967, pp. 497–498).

Salk published an account of his early trials at the Watson Home and the Post School in the *Journal of the American Medical Association* in March 1953. Rivers and others worked to dampen any expectations that a polio vaccine would soon be available for general use. Many polio scientists feared that if Salk's results were presented too positively, public pressure for an early field trial would increase, and the NFIP would then pressure scientists to proceed to a trial before they were ready. Salk did not content himself with reporting on his early results; he continued to inoculate children in western Pennsylvania as part of his effort to perfect his vaccine. By the early months of 1953, he had given the vaccine to an additional 5,000 children. As with the smaller group, the results were all positive. Antibody levels rose and no child developed a case of polio (Paul, 1971, p. 420).

As word began to spread that Salk was testing a polio vaccine in humans, the pressure on him and on the National Foundation for Infantile Paralysis that was funding his research increased substantially. To help dampen the growing expectation that a polio vaccine was imminent, Salk suggested to Basil O'Connor that he go on national radio to explain his experiments and to ask the American public to be patient. Salk appeared on CBS radio on March 26, 1953. He provided a brief summary of his work and the work of other polio researchers. In addition, he cautioned that patience was needed. He noted that "although progress has been more rapid than we had any right to expect ..., there will be no vaccine available for widespread use for the next polio season." He also noted, however, that "the amount of antibody induced by vaccination compares favorably with that which develops after natural infection." As David Oshinsky noted, this last statement meant that Salk's "killed-virus vaccine had worked just fine" (Oshinsky, 2005, p. 172). The news media put a very favorable spin on Salk's statement, implying that a vaccine would soon be available and giving credit to the American people who had contributed to this achievement by giving their dimes and dollars to the March of Dimes year after year. Many of Salk's colleagues in polio research were upset that Salk had discussed his experimental results before they were published in a medical journal, and they resented the attention he was receiving from the NFIP and the media.

Fifteen years after the establishment of the National Foundation for Infantile Paralysis, the organization was close to its goal of preventing polio. Funding from the NFIP had enabled scientists to understand the poliovirus and how it worked in the body to paralyze muscles. The work of Enders, Weller, and Robbins had made it possible to cultivate the large amount of virus needed to produce a vaccine. Salk's laboratory in conjunction with several others had demonstrated that there were only three types of poliovirus. And Salk, using techniques developed for the influenza vaccine, had developed a killed-virus polio vaccine that appeared safe in preliminary human trials. The final step would be to conduct a large trial to determine the vaccine's effectiveness in preventing polio.

10

The Polio Vaccines of Salk and Sabin

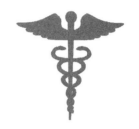

B y 1953, several scientists were working on developing a polio vaccine. Jonas Salk at the University of Pittsburgh had already tested his killed-virus vaccine on children and had demonstrated its safety and its ability to create or to increase the antibody level in children. Salk was using a method that had proven both safe and effective with influenza vaccine. Albert Sabin at the University of Cincinnati Medical School and Hilary Koprowski at Lederle Laboratories were both developing an attenuated live-virus vaccine. The vast majority of polio scientists believed that a live-virus vaccine was superior to a killed-virus vaccine, but the laboratories working on these vaccines needed additional time to work through all the problems of creating a safe and effective live-virus vaccine. Basil O'Connor at the National Foundation for Infantile Paralysis (NFIP) was pushing for a safe and effective vaccine as soon as possible. The previous year, 1952, had been one of the worst polio seasons in America with over 52,000 cases. Every additional year without a vaccine meant that tens of thousands of children, adolescents, and adults would suffer crippling paralysis from polio, and hundreds would die. But O'Connor's strong desire for an effective vaccine had to be tempered by the scientists' need for careful and rigorous testing of any possible experimental vaccine.

As Salk moved forward with his experimental vaccine, Basil O'Connor faced a problem within the National Foundation. The Immunization Committee clearly favored developing an attenuated live-virus vaccine that would be more effective and long lasting. Given that conviction, they were especially opposed to any early field trial of Salk's killed-virus vaccine. O'Connor and his scientific advisor Thomas Rivers decided that the members of the Immunization Committee were too invested in their own "special stake in the polio research" to be able to offer sound advice on the questions relating to the competing vaccines (Benison, 1967, p. 502). O'Connor decided to appoint a Vaccine Advisory Committee whose membership would not include any scientist "who had a personal stake in immunization research—whether it was Salk, Sabin, or anybody else for that matter" (Benison, 1967, p. 503). Several of the members of the Vaccine Advisory Committee were experts in public health, although both Dr. Rivers and Dr. Joseph Smadel were virologists. Some members of the Immunization Committee were upset that O'Connor had deprived them of a role in deciding whether the National Foundation would move ahead with the Salk vaccine or any other vaccine. O'Connor and Rivers, however, were confident that the new committee had members who could address the issues of polio vaccine without the divisions and tensions between the partisans of Salk and Sabin that had hindered decision making on the Immunization Committee. With this committee in place, O'Connor felt confident he would get the advice and support he needed regarding a possible field trial of a vaccine.

THE 1954 FIELD TRIAL OF THE SALK VACCINE

The Vaccine Advisory Committee debated the merits of a field trial of the Salk vaccine for much of 1953. There were several questions on the table. First, was the Salk vaccine ready for a large-scale field trial? Second, were the pharmaceutical companies capable of safely producing sufficient quantities of the vaccine? Third, what kind of trial would produce the best scientific results? Salk had proposed a trial in which one group of children was vaccinated, and a second control group was not. Both groups would be observed to see whether the vaccinated group had a lower rate of polio during the next polio season. Some members of the committee, especially Dr. Joseph Bell, an expert in child immunization who had been added to help plan the trial, wanted a double-blind placebo trial. This would be a trial in which neither the doctors administering the vaccine nor the volunteers receiving it would know whether the injected shot contained the vaccine or only an inert solution that looked like the real thing. This type of testing is generally considered better and more scientific because it eliminates any chance of bias on the part of individuals administering the experiment. Finally, they were not sure who should run the trial. They agreed that Salk should not run the trial of his own vaccine. Having an independent scientist unaffiliated with Salk's lab in charge of the field test would ensure its integrity and accuracy. That was important to Salk and the NFIP whether the test was successful or not.

Debates over a possible field trial of the Salk vaccine were heated both on the Vaccine Advisory Committee and within the National Foundation for Infantile Paralysis. A lot was at stake. First, of course, was the safety of the thousands of children who would be inoculated with an experimental vaccine. Second, the scientific reputations of the men running the test were on the line. Whatever the outcome, the field test needed to be fair and objective and to be perceived as fair and objective by both the medical community and the general public. Third, the reputation of the National Foundation for Infantile Paralysis was at stake. They had persuaded millions of Americans to contribute their dollars to the campaign against polio. If the Salk vaccine failed to protect children against polio or proved to be unsafe, or if the field trial was unsuccessful for any reason, the National Foundation would find it difficult to continue to raise the sums necessary to care for polio patients and to pursue its research program. The debates were so contentious that Harry Weaver, director of scientific research for the NFIP, left the organization in 1953, as did Dr. Joseph Bell. Before Bell left, however, he prepared a plan for the field trial that ultimately provided a blueprint for the actual trial. On November 13, the Vaccine Advisory Committee voted unanimously to recommend a field trial of the Salk vaccine (Oshinsky, 2005, pp. 174–181).

The success and credibility of the proposed field trial largely depended on the individual chosen to direct it. The NFIP needed an individual with an impeccable scientific reputation who was independent of both Salk and the National Foundation. In November 1953, Hart Van Riper, medical director of the NFIP, asked Dr. Thomas Francis to direct the field trial. Francis was on the faculty at the University of Michigan where he had distinguished himself in microbiology, internal medicine, and epidemiology. During World War II, Jonas Salk had worked in Francis's laboratory on developing an influenza vaccine. Salk learned from Francis the techniques of using formalin to create a killed-virus influenza vaccine, techniques he would later apply to the poliovirus. In 1947, Salk left Michigan to establish his own virology laboratory at the University of Pittsburgh. In the years following, Salk and Francis had relatively little contact as each pursued his separate lines of research. When he was asked to lead the field trial, Francis hesitated. Only after meeting with NFIP officials, including O'Connor, and carefully considering the challenges of the proposed trial did Francis agree to take charge.

Before he accepted responsibility for the field trial of the Salk vaccine, Francis required the NFIP to agree to several conditions. Francis demanded the freedom to run the trial without interference from the NFIP, although the National Foundation would pay all the expenses associated with the trial. He also wanted assurances that the NFIP would continue to support his own virus research during and after the trial. Finally, he insisted on having at least part of the trial run on a double-blind basis in which some children would be given the vaccine and a control group would be given a placebo. Neither the doctor administering the shot nor the individual being injected would know whether the shot contained the real vaccine. This was done to eliminate any possibility of bias in the experiment. Francis was also willing to have part of the trial run with observed controls in which one group of children was given the vaccine, and a comparable group was not but was observed to see whether any developed polio in the upcoming polio season. The Foundation and Salk accepted his conditions, and Francis agreed to run the trial in the spring of 1954 (Oshinksy, 2005, pp. 184–185; Paul, 1971, pp. 426–427).

Early in the planning stage, Dr. Francis decided that to be reliable the trial would have to involve large numbers of children. Because the actual incidence of polio in the population is relatively low, and because not every community experienced a polio epidemic every year, Francis needed large numbers of children scattered around the country to ensure statistically significant results. Francis and his team at the University of Michigan Poliomyelitis Vaccine Evaluation Center also had to decide which children to vaccinate. They ultimately decided there would be two different approaches in different communities involving first, second, and third grade students. For the part of the trial involving observed controls, second graders would be given the vaccine, and first and third graders would make up the observed controls. During the upcoming polio season both the vaccinated second graders and the unvaccinated first and third graders would be watched to see how many developed polio. For the double-blind part of the trial, first, second, and third graders would all receive an identical looking shot, but only half of the shots would actually contain the Salk vaccine.

Several considerations went into deciding in which communities the trial would be held. They wanted communities that represented the diversity of America, including rural, suburban, and urban locations. The planners focused on cities and counties of 50,000 to 200,000 populations because they would be easier to organize and manage. They also needed to identify counties that had the highest incidence of polio between 1948 and 1952 and were thought to be at high risk for another polio epidemic. The scientists hoped that in these counties they would find "the widest differences in 'attack rates' between those who would get the real vaccine and those who wouldn't. Furthermore, if the vaccine were proved to be even moderately effective, its use in high-risk counties would likely save more children from polio." Eventually, Francis and his colleagues chose "211 counties in 44 states—127 counties using observed controls and 84 using injected controls" (Oshinsky, 2005, p. 187). Approximately 1.3 million children would eventually participate in the largest vaccine trial in American history, either as recipients of the vaccine or as part of a control group.

Dr. Francis and his colleagues at Michigan, along with the NFIP, faced a daunting task in the early spring of 1954. The trial had to be organized; over 600,000 sets of vaccine had to be manufactured and purchased; thousands of local volunteers, including doctors and nurses to give the shots, had to be secured; and record-keeping for every child participating had to be established. As one participant noted at the time, "Our basic problem was to get three doses of [polio] vaccine or control solution into the arms of approximately 650,000 schoolchildren ... and keep accurate records on all involved in the trial" (Oshinsky, 2005, pp. 188–189).

Dr. Francis was responsible for running the trial and for analyzing the results, but the National Foundation was deeply involved as well. It paid for almost all aspects of the trial, a responsibility that strained even the NFIP's well-earned reputation for raising substantial sums of money. In addition to the $54 million raised during the annual January appeal, the NFIP conducted a supplemental campaign in August 1954 to raise an additional $20 million. Parents needed to be educated about the trials and its risks since they were being asked to volunteer their children for the experiment. O'Connor's letter to parents tried to impress on them the importance of the trial and the privilege their child would enjoy by becoming a "polio pioneer."

Instead of asking parents to give their permission for their child to participate, the form O'Connor devised phrased the permission as "I hereby request." Parents were assured that the Salk vaccine could not cause polio and had previously been tested safely on over 5,000 volunteers, including Salk and his family. The point of the trial was "to determine whether the vaccine, *already proved safe*, will give adequate protection against paralytic polio" (Oshinsky, 2005, pp. 190–191). In addition to convincing parents to volunteer their children for the trial, the NFIP had to find thousands of volunteers to administer the vaccine. Melvin Glaser, who coordinated the trial for the NFIP, estimated that "approximately 14,000 school principals, 50,000 classroom teachers, 20,000 physicians and 40,000 nurses would be needed." Another quarter of a million volunteers were needed to carry out all the logistical and other tasks of setting up the injection sites in schools and insuring that all the necessary equipment was in place on the appointed date (Oshinsky, 2005, p. 190).

Supplying adequate vaccine for the trial also proved to be difficult. Making the vaccine safe by inactivating the virus required manufacturers to follow Salk's recipe and procedures exactly. Each batch of potential vaccine was tested three times, first by the pharmaceutical company, then by Salk's laboratory, and finally by the Public Health Service. During practice runs only two drug companies, Eli Lilly and Parke-Davis, proved they could consistently manufacture safe quantities of the Salk vaccine. They provided all the vaccine used in the trial (Oshinsky, 2005, pp. 92–93).

In spite of the magnitude of the task of preparing for the trial, by April 1954, both Dr. Francis and the NFIP were ready to begin inoculating children. The National Foundation's Vaccine Advisory Committee voted unanimously on April 25 to proceed with the trial. Shortly after their vote was taken, the U.S. Public Health Service also approved the trial. Most parents were also

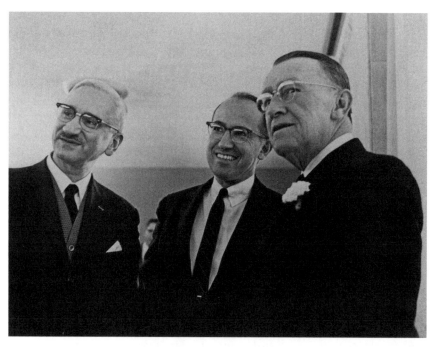

Three central figures in the development of polio vaccines: Dr. Albert Sabin, developer of the oral live-virus vaccine (left); Dr. Jonas Salk, developer of the killed-virus vaccine (center); and Basil O'Connor, president of the National Foundation for Infantile Paralysis that funded the research that led to the development of the two successful vaccines (right). (March of Dimes)

anxious to begin because they hoped that by enrolling their children as polio pioneers, they could protect them from the dread disease (Oshinsky, 205, p. 197).

The Salk field trial began in McLean, Virginia, where six-year-old Randy Kerr bravely received the first injection and became the nation's first polio pioneer. Over the next month or so, approximately 600,000 more grade-school children would be inoculated with the Salk vaccine. To receive full protection, each participating child needed to receive three shots, separated by a couple of weeks. Amazingly, 95 percent of those participating received all three shots (Oshinsky, 2005, p. 197). Every detail of the procedure had to be recorded. While doctors and nurses gave the injections, volunteers recorded the number of the vaccine batch, while others tossed out used needles and syringes and gave each child a lollipop for participating. There were numerous minor mishaps along the way, but no major problems emerged. Once all the shots were given, the paper records were collected and sent to the University of Michigan, where they would be analyzed following the polio season. All that Salk, Francis, O'Connor, and millions of parents could do now was wait—wait to see whether the vaccine provided adequate protection during the polio epidemics of that summer. That summer and fall, Francis was notified each time a child who participated in the trial died. Several hundred of the 1.3 million participants died, but most deaths were from other causes such as accidents, cancer, or pneumonia. Only about 5 percent of the deaths among participants were from polio (Oshinsky, 2005, p. 199). But until all the data were analyzed, no one would know how many cases of paralysis or deaths the vaccine had prevented.

Dr. Francis and his team at the University of Michigan faced a major challenge in evaluating the results of the trial. They had to analyze the records of all 1.3 million children who had participated and who experienced the 1954 polio season. They were looking for what didn't happen. That is, they were looking to see whether those children who received the Salk vaccine had a lower incidence of polio than those who were in the trial but who did not receive the shots. It took the team many months to tabulate all the statistics from the trial and then to analyze them to determine how effective the vaccine had been in providing protection against polio. Much of the data was tabulated by hand, although some of it was analyzed using an early computer. Francis insisted that no preliminary results be released or leaked, and none were, not even to Basil O'Connor, who was particularly anxious to know whether the vaccine he had pushed was effective. In March 1955, Francis notified O'Connor that the results had been analyzed and that he would need about a month to write his report. O'Connor offered Francis several dates on which to make the announcement, and Francis chose the last date, April 12. As O'Connor knew, that date was the tenth anniversary of the death of Franklin D. Roosevelt.

The questions of how and where to announce the results of the field trial were difficult to settle. Francis preferred to have the announcement made at a scientific meeting so as to emphasize the science behind the vaccine and the trial. Salk wanted it to be made at the prestigious National Academy of Sciences in Washington. While O'Connor accepted the need to validate the trial scientifically, he was confident enough of the success of the trial that he wanted it announced in a more public way that would also point up the contribution of the National Foundation for Infantile Paralysis in funding the development of the vaccine. Since the trial had been evaluated at the University of Michigan, the university wanted the announcement to be made on campus to draw attention to its research capabilities. Dr. Francis agreed to make the announcement at the University of Michigan in the large auditorium of Rackham Hall.

The first individuals outside the Polio Vaccine Evaluation Center to learn the results of the trial included Jonas Salk and Basil O'Connor, who met with Thomas Francis at a breakfast preceding his presentation. The Vaccine Evaluation Center had prepared a packet of material for the press, including a summary of the report that was to be handed out shortly before Francis began his address. The press had agreed not to distribute the news until Francis started talking at 9:30 A.M. However, when the packets were distributed to some 150 members of the press about 9:15, the news that the vaccine was successful was too good to keep under wraps for even a few minutes. The pressroom was chaotic as journalists dashed for phones to relay the good news to newspapers, radio, and television.

Although the news was already reaching the nation when Thomas Francis stood at the podium in Rackham Hall, he did not deviate from his plan to deliver a detailed scientific address outlining the results of the field trial. He emphasized that the vaccine was safe, although its effectiveness varied somewhat from one batch to another. Where the trial had been conducted with observed controls, Francis found that the vaccine had been "60–80 percent effective against paralytic poliomyelitis, 60 percent against Type I poliomyelitis and 70 to 80 percent effective against Types II and III." Where the double-blind test had been conducted, the results were similar. In those areas the vaccination had been "80–90 percent effective against paralytic poliomyelitis; that it was 60 to 70 percent effective against disease caused by Type I virus and 90 percent or more effective against that of Type II and Type III virus." The raw numbers show dramatically how effective the vaccine was. In the double-blind study areas, 200,745 children were vaccinated and 201,229 received the placebo. Only 33 children who were vaccinated developed polio, while 115 children in the placebo group developed the disease. In the observed study areas, there were 38 polio cases among the 221,988 children vaccinated, while there were 330 polio cases in the 725,173 children who did not receive the vaccine but were observed (Oshinsky, 2005, pp. 203–204). The media quickly spread the word that the Salk vaccine was both safe and effective.

The next step was to license the vaccine for general use. On the afternoon of the Francis announcement, the Public Health Service, then a branch of the Department of Health, Education, and Welfare (HEW) of the U.S. government, convened a meeting in Ann Arbor of prominent polio scientists to make a recommendation concerning licensing the vaccine. The scientists quickly read through the Francis Report and material from the drug companies concerning the manufacture of the vaccine. Given the acclaim that the morning's announcement had received, the group felt pressured to approve the vaccine quickly. After two hours of consideration, the group, including a somewhat reluctant Albert Sabin, voted unanimously to recommend approval. Shortly thereafter, the secretary of HEW, Oveta Culp Hobby, approved the license for the Salk vaccine. During the months that Dr. Francis was analyzing the data, Basil O'Connor was so confident that the vaccine would be safe and effective he paid the drug companies to produce 9 million doses of the vaccine. Once Hobby gave her approval, those 9 million doses began to be shipped to doctors across the country for injection into the arms of the nation's schoolchildren.

In the weeks following the announcement in Ann Arbor, Jonas Salk was treated as a hero by a nation relieved that his vaccine had conquered polio. Salk received awards from a number of cities, states, and the federal government. Congress, for example, authorized a Congressional Gold Medal to recognize his achievement. Salk was only the second medical scientist to receive the award. Salk and his family were also invited to the White House on April 23 to meet President Dwight D. Eisenhower. The president thanked Salk and promised to share the discovery with the world. Salk also spoke briefly to thank those who had contributed to the achievement, including his own laboratory staff, which he had neglected to thank in Ann Arbor. But even as Salk was accepting the thanks of the nation, disturbing news about the safety of the vaccine began to emerge.

Only two pharmaceutical companies, Eli Lilly and Parke-Davis, had produced the vaccine used in the field trial. However, several other drug companies had manufactured some of the vaccine to be used in the general population once it had been licensed. In addition to Eli Lilly and Parke-Davis, vaccine from Cutter Laboratories, Pitman-Moore, and Wyeth Laboratories had been approved by the federal government for distribution and use. Growing and inactivating the poliovirus comprised a complex process. It required many steps to insure not only that the virus had been killed but also that it retained its ability to produce antibodies when injected into an individual. If not all the steps were properly completed, live poliovirus could remain in the vaccine and cause a case of vaccine-induced polio. Salk was confident that if manufacturers followed the procedures precisely, his vaccine was safe, but his confidence was soon shaken.

THE CUTTER INCIDENT

Beginning on April 25, disturbing reports of cases of polio following vaccination with the Salk vaccine began to reach public health officials in Illinois, California, and Washington, D.C. By the following day, officials knew that six children had been paralyzed following their vaccination and that all six had been injected with vaccine manufactured by Cutter Laboratories. William Workman, the director of the U.S. Laboratory of Biologics Control, which had licensed the Salk vaccine, became the center of an intense set of meetings to decide on a plan of action. In a late-afternoon meeting on April 26, Workman David Price, the assistant surgeon general, Alexander Langmuir, the chief epidemiologist with the Communicable Diseases Center (now the Centers for Disease Control and Prevention) in Atlanta; and others from the Laboratory of Biologics Control and the National Institutes of Health reviewed what they knew about the emerging crisis. Langmuir later recalled that "when we began to fill in the gaps I became as convinced as anyone could be at this stage that the cases were attributable to a common source, the Cutter vaccine. Each of the children had fallen ill a few days after inoculation. In each case, the first paralysis had occurred at the site of inoculation. No comparable outbreaks of polio seemed to be taking place among unvaccinated children in the same communities." In other words, it had to be the Cutter vaccine that had caused these six cases of polio (Offit, 2005, pp. 65–68).

Vaccine from the Cutter Laboratories had been among the vaccines licensed immediately following Thomas Francis's announcement in Ann Arbor. There had been at least two warning signs of trouble concerning the manufacturing process at Cutter Laboratories, but these signs had not blocked the license for the company. Bernice Eddy had inspected the Cutter Laboratories for the Laboratory of Biologics Control to see whether any lots of polio vaccine contained live poliovirus. She tested the vaccine on monkeys and discovered that vaccine from three of the six test batches submitted by the company had caused polio in these animals. She reported her findings to William Workman, her boss, but he chose not to tell the committee that eventually licensed the vaccine. These particular lots were never released to the public, but the fact that Eddy found live poliovirus in supposedly inactivated polio vaccine indicated that there were serious problems in Cutter's manufacturing process. Julius Younger, a key member of Jonas Salk's laboratory, also visited Cutter Laboratories just after the vaccine was licensed. Cutter had contacted Younger in San Francisco, where he had gone for a meeting, and asked him about difficulties with completely killing the poliovirus for the vaccine. Younger was appalled by what he saw on a tour of the facility. Live poliovirus was grown in a room where the inactivated vaccine was stored. The record keeping was sloppy, but even so it revealed that Cutter was not achieving the kind of inactivation that Salk's laboratory had established as necessary. When Younger returned to Pittsburgh he informed Salk of Cutter's difficulties and offered to write the Laboratory of Biologics Control about his concerns. Salk said he would write the letters, but, for whatever reason, never did. For the rest of his life, Younger was burdened by the knowledge that he had failed to sound a warning that could have saved many lives (Offit, 2005, pp. 62–65).

Initially, the group called together by William Workman to deal with the crisis could not agree on how to proceed. Alexander Langmuir wanted to recall all the Cutter vaccine immediately, but the others decided to wait a bit before taking such a drastic step. On the morning of April 27, the Surgeon General of the United States, Leonard A. Scheele, joined the deliberations. During a telephone conference, he received conflicting advice regarding a course of action. Scheele faced several choices. He could recall the lots of Cutter vaccine that appeared to have caused polio. He could recall all lots of vaccine manufactured by Cutter. Or he could do nothing, which carried the risk that more cases of vaccine-induced polio might emerge. Scheele also confronted the problem that he had no legal means to force Cutter to recall its vaccine. By mid-morning, Scheele decided the safest course was to recall all lots of the Cutter vaccine, and he asked the company to voluntarily stop distributing its polio vaccine and to recall all its vaccine from doctors, hospitals, and clinics. Shortly after receiving Scheele's request, Cutter Laboratories sent a telegram to all doctors, drug stores, and other health facilities that had received its vaccine asking them to stop injections immediately and to return all unused vaccine to Cutter Laboratories. Robert Cutter soon issued a press release stating that while Cutter vaccine had not been definitely proven to be the cause of these polio cases, the safest course was to remove the vaccine from the market at least temporarily.

Scheele issued his own press release that tried to reassure the public that there was "no cause for alarm" regarding the Salk vaccine (Offit, 2005, pp. 68–71, 77–79).

But even as these assurances went out, the number of polio cases associated with the Cutter vaccine grew. "By April 30, within forty-eight hours of the recall, Cutter's vaccine had paralyzed or killed twenty-five children: fourteen in California, seven in Idaho, two in Washington, one in Illinois, and one in Colorado." Salk issued a statement supporting the recall and an investigation in the cause of the polio cases associated with the Cutter vaccine. His wife remembered that he was "concerned; he was worried; he was anxious; he was depressed" (Offit, 2005, p. 79). He knew his vaccine was good, effective, and safe, but he worried about what could happen in the manufacturing process if the companies did not follow all the protocols precisely or if they were sloppy in their handling of the poliovirus and the vaccine. The vaccine had been recalled quickly once the polio cases appeared, but by then some 380,000 children had already been vaccinated. No one knew how many additional cases would appear in coming weeks.

Langmuir was assigned the task of discovering the magnitude of what he called "The Cutter Incident." His task was complicated by the necessity to separate cases of wild polio that had coincidentally followed a vaccination from those caused by the vaccination. A case of polio could follow vaccination but not be caused by the vaccination if, for example, the child was already and unknowingly infected with the poliovirus at the time of her vaccination. Langmuir would employ for the first time the Epidemic Intelligence Service that he had helped establish in 1951 to help protect the United States from the threat of biological warfare. Ironically, its first use was to study "an inadvertent biological attack from a pharmaceutical company inside the country" (Offit, 2005, p. 85). Langmuir and his team of epidemiologists, physicians, medical officers, and health officials "gathered information about every case of polio that occurred in 1955: they determined the age, residence, and symptoms of every victim; they determined who had received polio vaccine and who had had contact with someone that had received polio vaccine; they determined who had gotten which specific lots of vaccine; they determined who was shedding polio virus from the intestines and what types of polio virus were being shed." They also compared the incidence of polio over the previous five years with that in 1955 (Offit, 2005, pp. 85–86).

Langmuir's team discovered that every case of polio that appeared to be caused by the Cutter vaccine came from two lots. For lots 19468 and 19764, "the incidence of paralysis was almost ten times greater than expected." The researchers discovered that "these two lots of Cutter's vaccine had paralyzed fifty-one children and killed five." The severity of these polio cases was also greater than that typically caused by wild poliovirus. Children who were vaccinated from these two lots were "more likely to be paralyzed in their arms, more likely to suffer severe and permanent paralysis, more likely to require breathing assistance in iron lungs, and more likely to die than children naturally infected with polio." This was largely due to the fact that Cutter had used the virulent Mahoney strain of polio to make its vaccine. According to Dr. Paul Offit, who has studied the Cutter Incident, "children infected with Cutter's vaccine were actually worse off than children attacked by natural polio virus" (Offit, 2005, p. 86). A study done in 1957 revealed that these fifty-six children were only a fraction of those harmed by the Cutter vaccine. It has been estimated that "at least one out of every three doses of contaminated lots of Cutter vaccine (120,000 doses) contained live polio virus; therefore, it is likely that abortive polio occurred in at least 40,000 children (one third of 120,000). Further, because abortive polio developed in only about one of every three children infected with natural polio, it is likely that all 120,000 children injected with Cutter's vaccine were injected with live virulent polio virus" (Offit, 2005, pp. 86–87).

Children inoculated with Cutter vaccine were not the only cases of polio associated with the bad vaccine. "Cutter's vaccine was at the center of a man-made polio epidemic." The CDC team eventually discovered "seventy-four unvaccinated family members that were paralyzed—half were parents and half were brothers and sisters of children that had received Cutter's vaccine" (Offit, 2005, p. 87). Many of these family members were "severely paralyzed; thirteen required iron lungs and five died from the disease." There were also cases outside these families that could be traced to the Cutter vaccine. These occurred among family friends or playmates of the children. "In the end, at least 220,000 people were infected with live polio virus contained in Cutter's vaccine; 70,000 developed muscle weakness, 164 were severely paralyzed, and 10 were killed. Seventy-five percent of Cutter's victims were paralyzed for the rest of their lives" (Offit, 2005, pp. 88–89).

Cutter's vaccine had the most severe problems, but it was not the only vaccine manufacturer to have difficulties inactivating the poliovirus. At a two-day meeting at the National Institutes of Health that began on April 29, government officials and others, including Jonas Salk, reviewed Cutter's procedures and met with representatives of the other manufacturers. Several of the other pharmaceutical companies admitted that they, too, had had problems inactivating the virus. This meeting produced no clear recommendation for the surgeon general, but a follow-up meeting on May 5 and 6 recommended that the vaccination program be halted until officials were certain it was safe to continue. On May 6, Surgeon General Scheele stopped the vaccination program, and the drug companies stopped the distribution of 3.9 million doses of the Salk vaccine. Following the announcement, William Workman visited each of the drug companies manufacturing the vaccine to inspect and review their procedures for inactivation. As he approved specific batches of the vaccine, they were released for use so that by May 14 over 1 million doses had been approved. Each of the companies, however, admitted that some lots of vaccine had contained live virus. The percentage of contaminated lots ranged from 21 percent at Parke-Davis to 2 percent at Pitman-Moore. Fortunately, unlike Cutter, none of these firms distributed vaccine that they knew was contaminated with live poliovirus. However, a study done during the summer of 1955 indicated that there had been a serious problem with one lot of polio vaccine manufactured by Wyeth Laboratories. There were an unusually high number of polio cases following inoculation from one lot of Wyeth vaccine, and the company recalled that particular lot. While government officials knew about the problem with Wyeth vaccine, it was never made public at the time (Offit, 2005, pp. 99–103).

After the government reviewed protocols, inspected manufacturing facilities, and required new safeguards, they allowed all of the pharmaceutical companies except Cutter to resume distributing the polio vaccine. Although parents were assured that the vaccine was now safe, many in the summer of 1955 were reluctant to have their children vaccinated. The summer of 1955 would be another epidemic year with more than 28,000 cases, many of which could have been avoided had the Salk vaccine been more widely used (Oshinsky, 2005, pp. 237–238). The vaccination program resumed slowly. Over 100 million doses were given in 1955 and 1956 without new problems emerging. Confidence in the vaccine gradually returned among the medical professionals and parents so that "between 1956 and 1961, 400 million doses of Salk's polio vaccine were administered in the United States without causing a single case of paralysis" (Offit, 2005, p. 120).

Wherever the Salk vaccine was administered in significant numbers in the late 1950s, the polio rates dropped significantly. As John Paul observed, "Once the painful episode of the Cutter incident had subsided, the triumph of the Salk-type vaccine became even more manifest." Polio rates in the United States dropped from 13.9 cases per 100,000 population in 1954 to just 0.5 in 1961 (Paul, 1971, p. 438). There were 38,476 polio cases in 1954, the year of the field trial, and only 1,312 in 1961 ("Incidence Rates," 1999, p. 3). In spite of all the difficulties, the Salk vaccine had set polio on a course of extinction in the United States and in several other countries where it was extensively administered.

DEVELOPMENT OF THE SABIN ATTENUATED LIVE VACCINE

Throughout the development of the Salk vaccine Dr. Albert Sabin retained his belief that an attenuated, or weakened, live poliovirus vaccine would be better and more effective than a killed-virus vaccine. An attenuated live-virus vaccine had been the preferred method of most polio scientists, but there were numerous difficulties to be overcome. Salk's vaccine used a method that had been extensively tried in other vaccines, especially influenza, and with the support of the NFIP, he was able to move more quickly to develop an effective vaccine. However, as early as the 1920s, a number of researchers had worked on a live-virus polio vaccine, but without much success. In the early 1950s, as Salk was beginning to test his vaccine, two polio researchers were working intensively on developing a live-virus vaccine. Dr. Hilary Koprowski conducted polio research at the pharmaceutical firm of Lederle Laboratories. Dr. Albert Sabin was on the faculty of the University of Cincinnati Medical School. Koprowski's research was largely supported by the drug company, but Sabin received substantial grants from the National Foundation to support his work. Although Basil O'Connor clearly believed that Salk would produce a workable vaccine sooner and supported him accordingly, he also saw the promise in Sabin's work and ensured that he was adequately funded (Oshinsky, 2005, pp. 243–244).

There were several theoretical advantages of a live-virus vaccine over an inactivated vaccine. Salk's trials had clearly shown that an inactivated vaccine would produce protective antibodies. However, there were some disadvantages to this approach as "immunity was not speedily produced, particularly in the very young, nor was it always long lasting." Booster shots, perhaps even annually, were necessary to ensure continued immunity to polio. There were also some advantages to an attenuated live-virus vaccine. First, since it was given by mouth, it mimicked a case of wild polio by establishing in the intestines a very weak case of polio that stimulated the body to produce protective antibodies. As Dr. John Paul observed, "The immune state was comparable to that following natural inapparent infection with 'wild' virus." In addition, immunity is stimulated within days rather than months, which meant that this vaccine could be used to halt an ongoing epidemic. Finally, administering the vaccine through the mouth on a sugar cube or a drop of liquid was easier than giving shots. In the late 1950s, however, concerns lingered about the safety of a live-virus vaccine. After all, you had to weaken the virus sufficiently so it could not cause paralytic polio yet keep it strong enough to stimulate the body's immune response (Paul, 1971, pp. 451–452). Both Koprowski and Sabin focused on finding ways to reliably weaken the poliovirus for use in a live-virus vaccine.

Sabin weakened poliovirus by infecting monkey tissue with a sample of the virus. Once the infection had taken and the virus had grown, Sabin then took virus from that sample and used it to infect yet another sample of monkey tissue. Each time he did this the virus was weakened, and he continued the process until he believed the virus was sufficiently weak so that it would not cause a case of paralytic polio but would still stimulate antibodies. He first demonstrated the safety of the weakened virus by injecting it into the spinal cord of chimpanzees. Sabin was convinced that if the weakened virus did not cause polio in these chimpanzees, it would be safe to use in humans. But he also needed to test it in humans. In early 1954, Sabin sought to test his vaccine on children institutionalized with mental illness, much as Salk had tested his vaccine. However, the NFIP, which was funding Sabin's research, refused to approve such a trial. In late 1954 and early 1955, Sabin secured permission from the NFIP to test his vaccine on 30 adult Ohio prisoner volunteers. The volunteers were promised $25 and a slight reduction in their sentences. After testing the blood of potential volunteers, Sabin chose thirty prisoners who had no antibodies to polio. While there was some risk to the trial, it went well. "All thirty prisoners developed antibodies to the three virus strains, and no one took ill" (Oshinsky, 2005, p. 246).

Hilary Koprowski tested his live-virus vaccine in Northern Ireland in 1956 at the invitation of Dr. George Dick, a virologist in Belfast. The investigators and their children were vaccinated before proceeding to the general population. However, problems quickly developed. When researchers tested the stool samples of children who had been vaccinated with Koprowski's vaccine, they discovered that the virus had regained its strength. And when they injected this virus that had passed through the children into monkeys, it caused paralytic polio in the animals. Dr. Dick immediately stopped the trial. Soon thereafter, Koprowski left Lederle Laboratories to take a position at the Wistar Institute in Philadelphia.

By 1956, Sabin had made considerable progress in developing his vaccine. That year, a delegation of physicians from the Soviet Union visited the United States to study how this country dealt with polio. Polio had become a serious problem in the Soviet Union, and they were looking for a vaccine to end the epidemics. The Soviet scientists visited the laboratories of both Jonas Salk and Albert Sabin. The visit to Sabin's lab went particularly well. Shortly thereafter, Sabin received an invitation to visit the Soviet Union, and he spent a month there visiting research facilities and making the case for his vaccine. Dr. Mikhail Chumakov, the head of the Polio Research Institute in Moscow, had to decide whether to use a version of the Salk vaccine or to try the new and largely untested Sabin oral vaccine. Because of some of the difficulties associated with the Salk vaccine and because Sabin and Chumakov had developed a good working relationship, the Soviets decided to use the Sabin vaccine. The Russians inoculated over 10 million children in 1959 using the new vaccine. Unlike the 1954 Salk field trial, this was not a carefully constructed experiment with controls and double-blind procedures. In the estimation of the Soviets, the vaccination program had gone so well that they soon decided to vaccinate all Russians under the age of 20, some 77 million children and adolescents. Given the Cold War animosities of the time, Sabin and others were concerned that the Russian results would not be taken seriously in the United States and among its allies. Dr. John Paul from the Yale Poliomyelitis Unit suggested that the World Health Organization, which was affiliated with the United Nations, send a reputable scientist to examine the Soviet program and write a report. He also suggested that his colleague Dr. Dorothy Horstmann would be an ideal candidate (Oshinsky, 2005, pp. 251–253).

Dr. Horstmann spent six weeks in the Soviet Union in 1959 studying the procedures and results of the Russian program. Horstmann's report was generally approving of the Soviet program of inoculation with the Sabin vaccine. She concluded that the Sabin vaccine was safe and effective, and that in the Soviet Republics where it had been administered, there was a "marked reduction of cases in 1959." Although she apparently had some reservations because of the incomplete data she was given, Horstmann's generally positive report was significant in validating the success of the Russian experiment with the Sabin vaccine (Oshinsky, 2005, pp. 253–254).

The apparent success of the Sabin trial program in Russia raised questions about whether—or when—the new vaccine would be available in the United States. Albert Sabin extolled the benefits of his oral vaccine at scientific meetings, but he had competition. The Salk vaccine was still in widespread use in the United States as the only licensed polio vaccine and, in the years since 1955, it had significantly reduced the polio rates in the country. There were also two other oral vaccines in the competition. Hilary Koprowski had continued his polio research after moving to the Wistar Institute and had tested his vaccine in the Belgian Congo in central Africa. Herald Cox had taken over the polio research at Lederle Laboratories after Koprowski left and had tested an oral vaccine in South America. In 1960, both Sabin and Cox ran small trials in the United States. Sabin inoculated almost 200,000 people in Hamilton County, Ohio, which included Cincinnati, while Cox ran a trial in Dade County, Florida, involving 400,000 subjects. Following the trials, the U.S. surgeon general approved the Sabin vaccine for manufacture in the United States, while denying approval for the Cox and Koprowski vaccines for failing to meet safety standards. There were many discussions in these years involving polio researchers, the NFIP and Basil O'Connor, the surgeon general, and representatives from the CDC and the National Institutes of Health regarding the choice of a polio vaccine for the United States. Jonas Salk, Basil O'Connor, and the NFIP strongly argued for the continued use of Salk's inactivated vaccine. Sabin and many other virologists and polio scientists urged the medical profession and the federal government to adopt the oral vaccine as the standard preventive against polio. In part, it was an important scientific debate about the relative merits and disadvantages of the two vaccines, but it also got caught up in the competition among men such as Salk, Sabin, and O'Connor with strong personalities and egos (Oshinsky, 2005, pp. 261–265).

In 1961, pressure to adopt the Sabin vaccine increased when the American Medical Association (AMA) voted to discontinue use of the Salk vaccine once the Sabin oral vaccine was licensed and available for use. Salk protested to the AMA and to the surgeon general of the United States, but he was unable to change minds. Later that year, Sabin's Type I oral vaccine was licensed for general use, and Type II and III would be licensed in 1962. As David Oshinsky has written, "By 1963 the battle for supremacy was over. The Sabin vaccine was in, approved by the government and endorsed by the AMA" (Oshinsky, 2005, p. 267). Public health officials soon mounted what they called "Sabin Sundays" in which all Americans, children and adults alike, were urged to come to the clinics to receive the Sabin vaccine. Even individuals who had received the Salk vaccine and who had had polio were urged to line up for the sugar cube containing the drop of fluid with the vaccine. Those who had received the Salk vaccine were encouraged to get the Sabin vaccine because it appeared to convey life long protection without the need for booster shots. Those who had had polio were urged to take the Sabin vaccine to protect themselves because having had one type of polio did not provide immunity against the other two. For the next thirty years, the Sabin polio vaccine would be used almost exclusively in the United States and in many other countries, bringing the polio rate almost to zero. The only downside to the widespread use of the Sabin oral attenuated vaccine was the possibility of a vaccine-induced case of polio. Because the virus was still alive in the Sabin vaccine, on rare occasions it caused a case of polio in an individual who received it or among his or her intimate contacts. In time, public health officials would reconsider the commitment to the Sabin vaccine, but for more than three decades it was the primary weapon against the crippling disease. The goal of Franklin Roosevelt and Basil O'Connor to wipe out polio had become a reality in the United States and most of the world by the end of the twentieth century.

11

Living with Polio

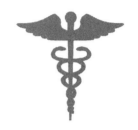

The success of the Salk and Sabin polio vaccines virtually eliminated polio as an epidemic disease in North America and Europe by the early 1960s. Polio began to recede from public memory to become simply one of many diseases against which children were vaccinated before they were school age. Polio, however, was much harder to forget for the hundreds of thousands who had been paralyzed by the disease in the decades preceding the wide distribution of the vaccines. The children, adolescents, and adults who had suffered from the disease had to find ways to live with polio. Once their rehabilitation was completed, virtually all polio survivors, even those dependent on iron lungs to breathe, returned home. Once home, polio survivors and their families had to learn to live well with a disability. That might mean altering the house or adjusting family responsibilities. Following this period of adjustment, the polio survivors had to begin to re-enter the worlds of school and work. They had to learn how to negotiate an often inaccessible world full of physical barriers such as stairs. Perhaps they had to adjust their future plans to accommodate their impairments. They also had to face the psychological challenges of living with a permanent disability. By and large, they succeeded in living full, rich lives, but it was never easy.

When polio survivors returned home from the rehabilitation hospitals, they often faced additional outpatient rehabilitation and sometimes surgery. Many went home with prescribed exercises that required the assistance of family members or perhaps a visiting nurse. Many polio survivors underwent surgery to try to correct deformities. Most surgeons waited to perform surgery until they were certain that no further improvement was possible through physical therapy. Since it could take up to two years for polio survivors to reach maximum function through physical therapy, surgery, if necessary, usually occurred two to ten years following the acute disease. These surgeries interrupted the survivors' recovery and return to something resembling a normal life, but they often prevented additional deformities or provided increased functionality.

After all the outpatient rehabilitation was completed and the last surgery was endured, polio survivors' physicians often told them that their condition was stable. Whatever remaining impairments they had would not get worse. That was reassuring news as it meant patients would not have to make adjustments to an increasing disability, unlike individuals with multiple sclerosis or muscular dystrophy whose disability worsened over time. Many polio survivors did experience a long period of stability, often several decades, but some twenty-five to thirty years after their illness many also began to experience new weakness, pain, and fatigue. In time, this condition came to be known as post-polio syndrome. As they aged, polio survivors discovered that their impairments did worsen, and they were forced once again to make adjustments to these new challenges. Living a long life with polio turned out to be more complicated than patients or physicians imagined during the height of the polio epidemics.

Polio survivors faced two challenges on returning home. First, there was the difficulty of getting around homes that were not handicapped accessible. Second, there was the challenge of reintegrating oneself into the life of the family. Before polio struck, these individuals had been healthy, active members of the family. They returned home changed both physically and psychologically. They had survived a serious illness, been paralyzed, and undergone extensive physical therapy often lasting weeks or months. They had been away from home for months, sometimes years. The family also faced the challenge of learning how to welcome their son, daughter, father, or mother back into the family's daily life. It took adjustments on both sides, and even if the process did not always go smoothly, most polio survivors did find a warm welcome on their return.

The first physical barriers that polio survivors encountered were in their own homes. Most houses in the mid-twentieth century had staircases, narrow halls and doorways, and slippery floors. Rural families sometimes still relied on outhouses. All these were difficult or impossible to negotiate in a wheelchair or with braces and crutches. Some families made substantial alterations to accommodate a son or daughter's disability, but most made no changes or only minor ones. When twelve-year-old Arvid Schwartz returned to his family's Minnesota farmhouse, he faced a steep winding stair to his upstairs bedroom. His father had gotten a two-by-two piece of lumber to fasten to the wall as a railing, but that was the only concession to his son's disability. His family expected him to learn how to get up and down stairs on his crutches and braces. As he recalled, "There weren't any aids, you just had to figure out how you were going to make this work" (Seavey, 1998, p. 262). Fourteen-year-old Charles Mee discovered that the changes his parents had made to their home had been "carefully chosen, enough to help, not enough to get me accustomed to living in any sort of specially constructed world. The parallel bars that I used to get in and out of the house were the only concession in the way of modification to the architecture of my home, and I stopped using them as soon as I could manage the four front steps of brick." Like many polio survivors, Mee recalls that he "learned to accept the world as it was and to adjust to it; that's the way I had been raised" (Mee, 1999, p. 121).

Family dynamics were often complicated by the polio survivor's return home. Any tensions between family members that existed prior to polio were often intensified by the need to provide care and to urge a son, daughter, or spouse to continue rehabilitation. Brenda Serotte remembers that her mother had never been particularly affectionate, but that her "mother's remoteness after I got polio distanced us further." From the day of her return, Serotte's mother "was loath to show any emotion regarding my physical struggles, nor did she give me any sympathy whatsoever, claiming later that she did not want to 'coddle' me." Her mother was "furious with me, with my illness, and with our whole situation in general." Serotte incorporated her mother's attitude into what she had already learned about being a polio survivor: "I knew I wasn't supposed to count on anyone's help to get around. The polio motto was, and always would be: Do it yourself, no matter how hard, no matter how long it takes. Mother must have known this, too, because she made no attempt to assist me then or in the difficult months that followed." Fortunately for Serotte, her "father was different; instinct told him when to step in, and he had no compunctions about helping me when I really needed it" (Serotte, 2006, pp. 141–142).

Richard Maus experienced a particularly difficult return home. He had polio in rural Minnesota in 1939, when he was only four months old. Two months later his parents took him to Gillette State Hospital in St. Paul, where he stayed for nearly a year. Because of distance, farm responsibilities, and hospital visiting rules, his parents only saw him twice in all that time. When he was released after 314 days in the hospital, he no longer recognized his parents. His parents were pleased to have him home again, but Richard "screamed in terror" every time his parents approached him or tried to pick him up. They were strangers to the young boy. His father had an idea one Sunday when his wife was at church. As Maus said, "He went to the bedroom closet and found a white shirt and a washed-out, nearly white pair of slacks. He put these on and walked out to the kitchen. When he approached me, I eagerly put out my arms. I wanted Dad to pick me up." Richard's willingness to be picked up reassured his parents that he had been treated well at the hospital. They quickly decided "to dress like doctors and nurses until I learned to accept them again. It took a few days" (Maus, 2006, pp. 8–9). As he grew, Maus had other difficulties with his family. He was repeatedly hospitalized for various surgeries but soon realized that "no one at home ever asked about my stay at the hospital. Not a word. If I brought it up, my family changed the subject. It made me feel as if I had done something that embarrassed them" (Maus, 2006, p. 63). In his early teens, Maus even contemplated suicide, but he decided to stay around for the sake of his dog Rex (Maus, 2006, pp. 76–77).

The families with a child or spouse in an iron lung faced the greatest challenges. Many polio survivors dependent on iron lungs or other respiratory machines to help them breathe returned home, but it was never easy. Families had to take on the primary responsibility for their care, even when they had some outside help. Louis Sternburg was married with two children when he was stricken with polio. After many months in an iron lung, he was able to use a rocking bed for breathing assistance. This was a bed that rocked like a teeter-totter. When the head went up, gravity pulled the diaphragm down and the patient breathed in; when the head went down, gravity and the internal organs pushed down on the lungs and the patient breathed out. Sternburg and his wife Dottie had not expected the transition home to be easy, but they thought they could manage. However, it proved to be even more difficult than they expected. They had the partial assistance of an aide, but Dottie Sternburg "learned all the slow and complicated details of nursing a paralyzed polio patient. She fed me and bathed me and dealt with bottles and bedpans, and massaged pressure points and changed my position constantly." In addition to caring for her husband, she also had to care for their two young children and keep the household running (Sternburg, 1986, pp. 75–76). They managed for many years, and while it became more routine and the children learned to help as they grew older, it was always difficult.

Even when the family member did not require around-the-clock care, families were still enlisted to assist with prescribed exercises and with those activities that paralyzed muscles made impossible. Most polio survivors needed to continue their physical therapy on their return home. Many went to outpatient therapy several times a week, but families took over on other days. Doctors sent Grace Audet home after seventy-nine days in the hospital. She went home with "a lot of muscle weakness," particularly in her upper body and with a "rather strenuous exercise program." Her father rigged up a temporary weightlifting apparatus to help her strengthen her muscles. Initially, her exercises took three and a half hours every day. After six months, she could raise her right arm for the first time since polio struck. When she returned to school full-time, her exercises were reduced to about two and a half hours daily. She followed this regime for several years (Sass, 1996, p. 251). These exercises and the muscle stretching that accompanied them were often painful, especially in the early stages, and often reduced children to tears and crying out in pain. But most parents persisted in spite of the physical and psychological pain because they knew that was the only way for their child to gain maximum function.

Painful exercises were not the only thing that tested the endurance of polio survivors. Orthopedic surgeons generally preferred to wait to operate to correct deformities until they were certain that patients had gained all they could through physical therapy. With children, they also preferred to wait until adolescence when the child had achieved much of his or her growth. Several types of surgery were common for individuals who had had polio, although each operation was unique depending on the particular muscles affected. Surgeons often fused joints, such as ankles, to give the patient greater stability. Other surgeons transplanted muscles and tendons to do the work of muscles paralyzed by polio. This might give an individual the ability to close his fist to pick up a glass, or perhaps the ability to write. Spinal fusions were perhaps the most dramatic of the polio surgeries. These were done to correct scoliosis or spinal curvature. Scoliosis was caused when muscles in the torso were paralyzed or weakened on one side, which pulled the spine out of alignment. Left untreated, spinal curvatures could impair breathing and the ability to function. Before a spinal fusion, surgeons used some device, perhaps a flexible cast or traction, to straighten the spine. They then fused all or some of the vertebrae to maintain a straight spine. These surgeries often involved several weeks of straightening before the surgery and a long recovery in a body cast following the operation.

Orthopedic surgery is never easy, but teenagers found these surgeries particularly difficult. It often had been several years since their rehabilitation had ended, and they were just beginning to feel comfortable and adjusted in high school. Suddenly, they were pulled back into the world of hospitals and pain and away from their friends. Dorothea Nudelman recalled what it was like to be sixteen and back in the hospital for her second surgery: "The hospital was like summer camp for polios. Surgeries were planned. You booked a spot in advance." She thought she "could handle it. After all it was my second surgery. . . . I had hospitals down cold by now." But it was more difficult than she had expected. "The worse part, though, was going into the hospital feeling healthy and pretty and then experiencing pain and bodily violation in a way that was totally debilitating. It was like losing it all over again, only this time I wasn't a little kid anymore" (Nudelman, 1994, pp. 134–135). Adolescents, much to the surprise of the surgeons, often had considerable say in whether a surgery was to take place. Parents rightly reasoned that their son or daughter would have to live with the results and that they were mature enough to make a good decision. For example, Charles Mee's surgeon recommended an operation that would fuse his thigh so that it would point straight down. This would have made his leg more stable for walking, but it also meant that he would never be able to sit normally again. His parents asked him if he wanted to proceed, and when he had reservations, the surgery was called off (Mee, 1999, p. 178).

In spite of the challenges of continued therapy and occasional surgery, most polio survivors made a good transition home. Home-cooked meals were a special treat after hospital food, and sleeping in one's own bed was a special delight. Families generally expected their children with polio to participate in family responsibilities to the extent that they were able. Parents were advised not to coddle or spoil their children with polio, and most did not. Gail Bias lived on a farm and her parents expected her to do chores along with her siblings. Baling hay was about the only thing she couldn't do. Stanley Lipshultz couldn't do many of the outdoor chores on the family's farm, so he "washed more than my fair share of dishes and did other chores that did not require a lot of walking" (Wilson, 2005, p. 171).

Siblings and neighborhood friends often helped young polio survivors adjust to living with their disability. Don Kirkendall's brothers tied him in a buggy so he could accompany them when they went hunting. His paralyzed legs didn't impair his ability to shoot. I remember that neighborhood baseball games made accommodations for my inability to run. Sometimes I would bat, and a teammate would run the bases. Other days I was the permanent pitcher or, perhaps, the umpire. Since so many childhood games in the 1940s and 1950s were improvised, there was usually a way to include the children who had had polio. That is not to say that there weren't difficult moments. Children can be cruel, and sometimes the polio survivors were taunted for their limps or their hunchbacks.

Going out in public was often difficult for polio survivors, especially at first. Sidewalks were often uneven or non-existent, and steps and curbs presented other barriers. Until their full strength returned and they learned to walk confidently on braces and crutches, polio survivors often fell. The embarrassment of falling in public sometimes hurt more than any real physical pain. Survivors in wheelchairs faced many challenges in an era before curb cuts, ramps, and automatic doors. Jan Little recalls that in the 1950s "wheelchairs were associated with old or sick people" and "being in a wheelchair carried a fair amount of shame." After her parents had taken her on an outing, they were criticized for "taking a child like that out in public" (Little, 1996, p. 10).

Most young polio survivors were eager to return to school, partly because they missed their friends and the routine, but also because being back in class meant things were returning to normal. However, many grew anxious as the first day of school approached. Would they be able to keep up with the work? After all, many had missed weeks, sometimes months, of formal schooling. Although rehabilitation centers had classrooms and tutoring was sometimes done at home, many returning polio survivors worried about keeping up with their classmates. Returning polio survivors were also concerned about their reception. They had changed in the intervening months, and many returned reliant on braces and crutches or a wheelchair for mobility. Patients also worried about negotiating the schools of mid-Twentieth-century America. Most older schools had steps up to the front door and several floors of classrooms. Few schools had elevators. Some schools moved classes to accommodate students in wheelchairs, but survivors on crutches were often expected to negotiate the stairs. Sometimes friends carried a classmate and his wheelchair from floor to floor.

Young polio survivors with respiratory paralysis who were dependent on a respirator to breathe often did not return to school. Many school districts had provisions for teaching homebound students, but these programs seldom matched the quality of in-class instruction. When Mark O'Brien returned home, he was able to use a chest respirator instead of an iron lung and could spend several hours outside the respirator during the day. However, he was still unable to go to school. Initially, the school district provided him with a teacher who went to his home a couple of times a week. In grades five and six, he attended class by speakerphone, although it was difficult to hear what was happening in the classroom. For high school, O'Brien was again taught by teachers sent to his home by the school district. He eventually took a test and received his general equivalency degree. O'Brien thought he received a "pretty good education because I was working one-on-one with them and I was very eager to please them" (O'Brien, 2003, pp. 37, 41; Seavey, 1998, p. 110).

Jan Little's parents fought tenaciously to persuade the school district to allow her to return to high school in her wheelchair. Initially, the superintendent of schools refused because it was a multi-story building, and it was "inconvenient" to rearrange classes. He also thought it was a waste to educate a child who was permanently crippled, and it would depress the other students to have to look at Little every day. The high school principal did provide teachers to go to her home to teach her for the first two years of high school. By the time she was a junior, the district had built a new one-story high school, but it was still a struggle for her to get admitted. She and her parents had to promise not to ask for any special accommodations. Because none of the bathroom doors were wide enough for the wheelchair, Little had to go through the entire day without access to the bathroom. In spite of the negative attitudes of one teacher, Little enjoyed being back in school. She even joined the debate team, and as she recalls, "Roger and Bill, my debate team partners, managed to carry me up and down stairways in schools all over southeastern Wisconsin and only drop me a little way one time" (Little, 1996, pp. 12–15). Little's experience is good evidence that not all the barriers polio survivors encountered as they resumed their lives were physical ones.

Physical education and dating posed two difficult challenges for polio survivors returning to high school. The physical impairments typical of polio made it difficult for them to run, exercise, or participate in games during gym. While some were excused from gym, PE teachers sometimes made it easier for polio survivors. Ed Sass, who had scoliosis, recalls that the gym teacher always assigned him to the team that wore T-shirts rather than bare backs, thus sparing him additional embarrassment (Sass, 1996, p. 103). Coaches sometimes invited students who could not play to become team managers. I was unable to march with the marching band, but the conductor always found ways for me to help him on the sidelines.

Dating also challenged many adolescent polio survivors. Many young men were reluctant to ask a classmate out on a date for fear that she would reject him because of his disability. And many young women feared they would never be asked out because of their paralysis. The only thing that "really bothered" Arvid Schwartz about high school was his failure to date. As he later recalled, "I guess I figured that no one would want to go out with me, so I didn't have a girlfriend." He only began to date in college (Sass, 1996, p. 150). Gail Bias remembers that she didn't like to dance in high school because of her limp and feeling that people would "stare" and "gawk" at her on the dance floor. Bias commented that "all teenagers are self-conscious, but when you have some physical disability, it really magnifies that self-consciousness" (Sass, 1996, p. 82). Others were more successful in finding dates. Irving

Zola's friends arranged a date for him after he returned to Boston Latin, and, fortunately, the young woman accepted. He didn't want "to think about what would have happened if the girl had refused the date and my later advances." Charles Mee dated a cheerleader for a while in high school, and, since she was "pretty and energetic," she also brought him "into the mainstream with her" (Wilson, 2005, pp. 188–189).

Because polio limited what many survivors could do physically, many young men and women who had polio attended college to improve their chances of finding employment. Teenagers who had not been particularly serious about their studies in high school put more effort into their education following polio. Some, especially from the working class, admitted that they would never have considered college if they had not had polio. Since polio did not impair intellect or cognition, continuing their education made sense for many polio survivors. However, guidance counselors and admissions officers often underestimated polio survivors and made it difficult for them to go to college. In addition, in the 1950s and 1960s, colleges made few if any accommodations for students with physical limitations. If they were admitted, polio survivors were expected to figure out how to make it work largely on their own.

State departments of vocational rehabilitation paid for the college costs of some polio survivors, but not all such departments responded favorably to the polio survivor's desire to attend college. Jan Little's high school guidance counselor advised against continuing her education because "no college or university would accept a person in a wheelchair as a full-time residential student" (Little, 1996, p. 15). Little eventually attended the University of Illinois in her wheelchair. Ed Roberts posed a bigger challenge for the University of California since he still needed to be in his iron lung for part of the day. Still, he was determined to go to the University of California, Berkeley. California's Department of Vocational Rehabilitation initially refused his request for aid because "spending money on Roberts would be wasted since it was 'infeasible' that he could ever work." The department eventually relented following news reports of its decision, but getting into the university also posed a challenge. One of the deans refused to admit him on the grounds that "we've tried cripples before and it didn't work." Roberts was admitted only after the university hospital agreed to allow Roberts to move his iron lung to the facility (Shapiro, 1993, pp. 44–45).

Problems did not end once these polio survivors arrived on campus. Except for a few places such as the University of Illinois, no college or university was prepared to accommodate a person in a wheelchair, much less an iron lung. Most institutions presented serious obstacles to students in wheelchairs or who used braces and crutches for mobility. For example, when David Kangas arrived at the University of Minnesota in the fall of 1955, he discovered that "the University wasn't accessible for a person in a wheelchair." He saw "steps all over the place." Unlike high school, where a group of friends carried him from floor to floor, here he had to rely on the good will of strangers to try to reach his classrooms. He lived off campus because none of the dorms was accessible. Kangas had a car with hand controls, but finding parking was difficult because there were no handicapped spaces. It took Kangas five years to graduate because he "had to drop so many classes." He "couldn't get to some classes enough because accessibility was such a problem" (Sass, 1996, pp. 66–67).

By the mid-1960s, when Ed Roberts attended Berkeley, things had gotten a little better. The state paid for Roberts's attendants, who assisted him with dressing and eating and in negotiating the campus. They had to figure how best to get from place to place and which were the most accessible entrances to buildings. Roberts eventually got a motorized wheelchair, which gave him greater independence. Newspapers covered Roberts's experience because it was so novel, and this coverage encouraged other significantly disabled students to apply to the university. Soon there were twelve men and women living in the student hospital and attending the university. They eventually called themselves "The Rolling Quads" and began to agitate for removal of the barriers to accessibility. This was the era of student protests on university campuses, and the Rolling Quads caught some of that spirit in making their own demands. They wanted curb cuts, accessible housing outside the infirmary, and other accommodations so they could live and study like students without disabilities. Berkeley responded to many of their demands, and by 1970 established the Physically Disabled Students Program to assist disabled students in adjusting to university life and to ensure that the university was more accommodating (Wilson, 2005, p. 191).

Finding work also posed significant challenges for polio survivors. There were, of course, the usual physical barriers, especially stairs, but the attitudes of the men and women doing the hiring were often bigger barriers to employment. Even during World War II, when there was a shortage of workers, polio survivors were turned away. Twenty-nine employers refused to hire Don Kirkendall, who used a wheelchair. As one employment agency official told him, "It is the wheelchair, Donald. Nobody seems to want to take the risk of hiring a man in a wheelchair, no matter how well he can do the job" (Kirkendall, 1973, pp. 135, 208–210). Although he had a license to teach, no school in the Chicago area would hire James Doherty because, as he later recalled, "My physical disability would prevent me from shepherding students out of the school to safety in the event of a fire." Doherty eventually found work with the State of Georgia and with the Social Security Administration, but he never taught (Doherty, 1997, pp. 40–41). David Kangas moved to California after graduating from the University of Minnesota to avoid the harsh winters. There, and later when he returned to Minnesota, he took civil service exams to work in state government. He took the exams because "back in the 1960s, if you were disabled, just getting any kind of job was a mammoth undertaking. If you could even get an interview, you were lucky. There was no affirmative action at all, and it quickly became apparent to me that in private industry, opportunities were virtually nonexistent." With the state civil service, "If you took the exam and got first, second, or third highest score, they would at least have to give you an interview" (Sass, 1996, pp. 68–69). In spite of the difficulties and the prejudice they faced, most polio survivors who were able to work did so. Only about 10 percent of polio survivors never worked following polio.

In the 1950s and 1960s, many married women did not work outside the home. Since a high percentage of female polio survivors married, large numbers of them had to figure out how to run a household with their disability. Some had counters or ironing boards modified so that they could work at them. Their children often took on the household responsibilities of washing clothes, washing dishes, and cleaning earlier than they might have otherwise. These women discovered that it wasn't the chores they could or could not do that defined their role as mothers and wives. It was, instead, the support they gave their husbands and the guidance they gave their children that were most important, and polio did not affect those important roles.

Polio survivors wanted nothing more than to return to their lives following their disease and rehabilitation. To do so they had to surmount a number of obstacles, including barriers to accessibility and the prejudices of school administrators and employers. But polio survivors were also determined. They had learned in rehabilitation that hard work and persistence produced results: they had regained muscle function and strength. When they returned to the worlds of school and work, those lessons were applied to gaining entry and overcoming prejudice. Not everyone succeeded, and some had to settle for less than they had hoped, but, by and large, polio survivors made their way in the world whether walking, riding in a wheelchair, or relying on braces and crutches.

Their experience with discrimination because of their disability led some polio survivors to become activists on behalf of disability rights. We have already seen how Ed Roberts and the Rolling Quads persuaded the University of California at Berkeley to make the institution more accessible and welcoming to students with disabilities. Roberts and his friends soon set their sights higher. They pushed the City of Berkeley to install curb cuts and make other changes to accommodate individuals with disabilities. In 1972, Roberts and his friends opened in Berkeley the first center for independent living. The independent living movement rejected the notion that people with disabilities were invariably dependent, and they viewed disabilities as the result of the barriers that society imposed on individuals with a wide variety of impairments. Roberts argued that "independence was measured not by the tasks one could perform without assistance but by the quality of one's life with help" (Wilson, 2005, p. 192). The independent living movement soon spread across the country with centers opening in many cities. Judith Heumann was initially denied a license to teach in New York because she used a wheelchair. While the decision was eventually overturned, the experience led Heumann into disability activism when she established Disability in Action to agitate for disability rights. Heumann later joined forces with Ed Roberts at the center for independent living in Berkeley. Roberts and Heumann would both have distinguished careers. Governor Jerry Brown of California appointed Roberts as director of the Department of Vocational Rehabilitation, the department that had once rejected his application for tuition aid on the grounds that he would never be able to work. Heumann eventually served as assistant secretary of education in the administration of President Bill Clinton. Polio survivors would also be important backers of the Americans with Disabilities Act that passed in 1990 and was signed into law by President George H.W. Bush.

POST-POLIO SYNDROME

As they embarked on their careers or began their families in the 1950s and 1960s, polio survivors expected to put polio behind them. Doctors had assured them that their condition would not worsen with time, and having learned how to live with their disabilities, they got on with their lives. However, polio had one last surprise—post-polio syndrome (PPS). Beginning in the late 1970s and early 1980s, polio survivors from the large epidemics of the 1940s and 1950s began to experience troubling new symptoms in the muscles that had been affected by the initial disease. They reported a wide variety of symptoms, but the major ones were new pain, new muscle weakness, and fatigue. As mentioned above, polio survivors were discovering that some twenty-five to thirty years after they had the disease their body was failing them again. Men and women who had gotten out of the wheelchair to walk with braces and crutches found themselves back in wheelchairs because their arm and leg muscles had gotten too weak to carry them. Others needed new braces, or perhaps a cane or a scooter for long distances. Dealing with the physical changes was difficult, but so too was confronting the associated psychological issues. It was difficult to become more dependent, to give up activities once taken for granted. Men and women who had adjusted to their original disability now found themselves disabled in new ways that challenged their sense of well-being.

Doctors in the early 1980s, when polio survivors first reported these distressing symptoms in large numbers, often dismissed the idea that this new pain, weakness, and fatigue had anything to do with the attack of polio decades earlier. Polio survivors were often told that they had been working too hard or that they were imagining the pain and weakness. Some were referred to psychologists and psychiatrists. However, the problem was in the bodies of the polio survivors and not their heads. In the mid-1980s, a group now known as Post-Polio Health International began to collect accounts of these physical problems from polio survivors. Under its then director Gini Laurie, the organization held several meetings of polio survivors and doctors that helped convince doctors that something indeed was happening to the bodies of polio survivors several decades after the attack of polio. Although post-polio syndrome is still not well understood by the medical profession, most physicians now accept that it indeed involves physical changes in aging survivors.

The current consensus on post-polio syndrome is that it involves changes in the nerves and muscles that were affected by the initial attack of polio. The onset of post-polio syndrome probably involves several factors. Factors that physicians have identified include normal aging and overuse of the nerves and muscles that remained following polio. The nerves and muscles that remained after polio often had to do extra work for the polio survivor to use his or her arms and legs or to breathe. This extra burden on these nerves and muscles may cause them to wear out faster than normally.

For a diagnosis of post-polio syndrome, patients must have one or more of the following symptoms: "new weakness, unaccustomed fatigue, muscular pain, new swallowing problems, new respiratory problems, cold intolerance, and new muscle atrophy" (Silver, 2001, p. 17). Because post-polio syndrome is a "diagnosis of exclusion," physicians settle on that diagnosis only after other possible causes for the symptoms have been eliminated. In addition to the symptoms listed above, polio survivors need to meet four additional criteria: "1. An individual must have a known history of polio. 2. The individual must have had some improvement in strength following the initial paralysis. 3. There must have been a period of stability (at least one or two decades) in which the individual had no new symptoms. 4. The individual must present with new symptoms that are consistent with PPS and not attributable to some other disease" (Silver, 2001, pp. 17–18). Not all polio survivors will experience the symptoms of post-polio syndrome, but all are at risk.

Leonard Kriegel began to develop post-polio syndrome almost forty years after he had polio as an eleven-year-old boy in 1944. Polio had paralyzed

Kriegel's legs, but he had learned to walk with braces and crutches and was proud of the fact that he didn't need to rely on a wheelchair. As a boy, he had learned to fall safely and to get up again unassisted. For almost forty years, Kriegel's strong upper body had propelled him through the streets of New York where he had become a professor of English. One night in 1983, he fell to the sidewalk and to his surprise was unable to get up without the assistance of accompanying friends. His friends blamed it on the wet pavement, but Kriegel knew better: "It had to do with a subtle, mysterious change in my own sense of rhythm and balance. My body had decided—*and decided on its own, autonomously*—that the moment had come for me to face the question of endings." It was Kriegel's first encounter with post-polio syndrome (Kriegel, 1991, pp. 16–17). As his symptoms progressed, Kriegel found himself using a wheelchair more and more, and, finally, all the time. As he reflected on the move back to the wheelchair, Kriegel observed that "getting back into the wheelchair was not the spiritual death I feared." Still, he wondered if he "made the move too early." Perhaps he still had "a few years of walking on braces and crutches left—no matter how difficult the effort." In the end, he concluded he had made the right decision after all (Kriegel, 1998, p. 45).

Nancy Baldwin Carter, like Kriegel, was surprised when she began to experience the initial symptoms of post-polio syndrome. For her, extreme fatigue was the first to appear. Her fatigue became so severe that she was forced to change jobs to one less demanding and more sedentary. It worked for a while, and then the fatigue returned: "Exhaustion blended into weakness that somehow produced pain." When it became unendurable, she sought medical help: "Doctor after doctor sent me down a useless path. I saw an unbelievable seven physicians, each one diagnosing his own specialty—the rheumatologist said I had arthritis, while the orthopedist was sure that poor posture was the culprit." It was not until she returned to Warm Springs, where she had been treated as a child, that a doctor diagnosed her problems as post-polio syndrome. Her family physician still didn't believe the diagnosis and suggested she see a psychiatrist. Carter was forced to stop working and to severely restrict her activities. However, she refused to admit she had become disabled: "I did not want to be disabled. The word itself was repugnant to me. . . . I may have been using a wheelchair, unable to complete household tasks, struggling with breathing and swallowing, but by God, *I was not disabled*" (Carter, 1998, pp. 221–222). Now, Carter spends much of her time in bed to conserve her strength and her weakened muscles, but she has also begun to come to terms with this new phase of living with her polio. As she has written, "I do what I can. I deal with today. If I'm still here by bedtime, it's been a good day. I am happy" (Carter, 2006, p. 221).

Following polio and rehabilitation, polio survivors generally tried to live lives that were not defined by polio and disability. Whether their polio-caused impairment was minor or severe, most wanted only to get back to the lives they left when they entered the hospital weeks or months earlier. They returned home and to school. Where they could, they returned to the jobs they had before polio, and where that was not possible, most found new ones. Polio survivors went to college and graduate or professional school. They became teachers, businesspeople, professors, doctors, homemakers, lawyers, and disability rights activists. They married and had families and tried to partake of the post–World War II American dream. By and large they succeeded. Some, of course, did not. Some died because of the damage polio had done to their respiratory system. Some were unable to find good jobs because of discrimination. But, aided by the perseverance, hard work, and patience learned in rehabilitation, most polio survivors built good lives in the decades following the disease. What they had not expected was post-polio syndrome. Its symptoms forced them to confront once again polio-related pain, weakness, and the inability to do familiar things. Over the years, many polio survivors have adjusted to the limitations of post-polio syndrome, just as they earlier adjusted to the limitations imposed by polio, but experiencing a new disability has been difficult. And many are left wondering what other surprises polio might have in store for them.

12

The Campaign to Eradicate Polio

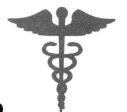

From the beginning of scientific research on polio in the early twentieth century, scientists and physicians sought a way to prevent or to cure the disease. Researchers such as Karl Landsteiner, Simon Flexner, John Paul, Dorothy Horstmann, John Enders, Jonas Salk, and Albert Sabin spent many hours in the laboratory and in the field trying to understand the virus that caused this crippling disease and to develop an effective vaccine against it. As we have seen, scientists had to overcome numerous challenges before they developed effective vaccines in the 1950s and 1960s. When polio research began, virology, the study of viruses, was in its infancy, and there were many false starts before Jonas Salk and Albert Sabin developed their effective and safe vaccines. These vaccines raised hopes that polio could be eradicated, but as with most developments concerning polio, eradication has proven to be more difficult than initially anticipated.

The Salk and Sabin vaccines quickly reduced the number of polio cases in the countries where they were used extensively. In the United States, for example, there were over 57,000 cases of polio in 1952, three years before the Salk vaccine was made available. The Salk vaccine reduced that number to 3,190 cases in 1960. Following the introduction of the Sabin vaccine in the early 1960s, the number was reduced to fewer than 100 cases per year by 1967

("Incidence Rates," 1991, p. 3). Similar declines occurred in other countries. Great Britain went from an average of 4,381 cases per year from 1951–1955 to 322 cases per year from 1961–1965. Czechoslovakia went from an average of 1,081 cases per year from 1951–1955 to no cases from 1961–1965 (Paul, 1971, p. 468). By the end of the 1960s, polio had been largely eliminated from North America, much of Europe, Australia, and New Zealand. Even in these areas, there continued to be a handful of cases each year where the Sabin oral vaccine was employed. Most of these cases were vaccine derived in individuals with weak immune systems, or where the weakened virus reverted to a virulent variety capable of causing paralysis. Polio, however, remained a serious threat in much of the developing world, where polio immunization was spotty and where other intestinal diseases reduced the effectiveness of the Sabin oral vaccines.

During the 1970s, world health officials took several steps toward reducing the annual toll of polio in those countries where it was still prevalent. In 1974, the World Health Assembly passed a resolution to create an Expanded Program on Immunization to increase the number of children vaccinated against common diseases including polio. Health officials also conducted lameness surveys in numerous countries during the 1970s seeking evidence of polio to determine the number of children paralyzed by the disease. When the surveys revealed widespread evidence of polio's destructiveness, many countries added the oral polio vaccine to their immunization programs. The battle against polio gained additional support in the 1980s. In 1985, the Pan American Health Organization (PAHO) began a campaign to eradicate polio from the Western Hemisphere. The same year, two United Nations agencies, the United Nations Children's Fund (UNICEF) and the World Health Organization (WHO), developed the Universal Childhood Immunization Initiative to reduce childhood mortality by increasing vaccination rates, especially in the poorer nations of the world. In 1987 and 1988, Rotary International, a service organization with members in many countries, raised nearly $250 million for programs to eradicate polio. Given the growing support for polio vaccination, the World Health Assembly in 1988 resolved to eradicate polio worldwide by the year 2000 (Global Polio Eradication Initiative, 2008, "The History").

The decade of the 1990s saw world health officials make additional progress toward their goal of eradicating polio. The most significant step occurred in 1991, when doctors recorded the last case of wild polio in North and South America. A young Peruvian boy, Luis Fermin Tenorio, came down with the last case in the Western Hemisphere acquired from wild poliovirus. Three years later, the health authorities declared the Western Hemisphere polio free, marking an important milestone in the effort to eliminate polio. During the 1990s, many nations in Africa and Asia instituted national immunization days to vaccinate as many children as possible. For example, in 1994, China held several National Immunization Days and vaccinated over 80 million children. China's immunization campaign was so successful that the last case of wild polio in China occurred in 1996. India held its first immunization days in 1995 and vaccinated over 87 million children. In the late 1990s, the campaign against polio accelerated. In both 1996 and 1997, over 450 million children were vaccinated during National Immunization Days in more than 90 countries where polio was still endemic. In a number of war-torn countries of Asia and Africa, cease-fires were arranged so that children could be vaccinated against polio and other diseases. Significant progress was recorded in 2000. That year, there were only 719 cases of wild polio recorded in the world, down from 350,000 in 1988 when the eradication program began. Over 550 million children were immunized against polio in 2000 (Global Polio Eradication Initiative, 2008, "The History").

When the eradication program began, doctors chose to use the Sabin or oral polio vaccine (OPV). There were four reasons doctors chose the OPV rather than the Salk or inactivated polio vaccine (IPV). First, because the OPV is given by mouth and passes into the intestines, it mimics cases of wild polio. It also fosters the development of antibodies in the intestine so that they are present when a child encounters the wild poliovirus. This means the OPV is more effective in stopping a polio epidemic. Second, the OPV is very easy to administer, and it is easy to train individuals in its administration. This made it easier to conduct the massive campaigns necessary to control polio. In 2001, for example, there were 10 million volunteer vaccinators. The IPV is more difficult to administer because it is given by an injection and requires skilled vaccinators. Third, the OPV is less expensive than the IPV, in part because the WHO and its partners were able to negotiate a special price for the developing world. Finally, the OPV immunizes children who do not directly receive the vaccine. Because the OPV is given by mouth and settles in the intestine, it is also shed in the stools of vaccinated children. This means that in conditions of poor sanitation, children who were missed on immunization days are likely to encounter and ingest the attenuated poliovirus shed by immunized children and thus acquire immunity as well (Seytre and Shaffer, 2005, pp. 114–115).

The effort to eradicate polio continued into the new century. Millions of children continued to be vaccinated, particularly in parts of Africa and Asia, where wild poliovirus was still paralyzing children. Some of the countries where polio remained, such as Afghanistan and Somalia, posed particular challenges because ongoing military conflict made it difficult to reach all children not yet immunized. By 2002, endemic polio could be found in only seven

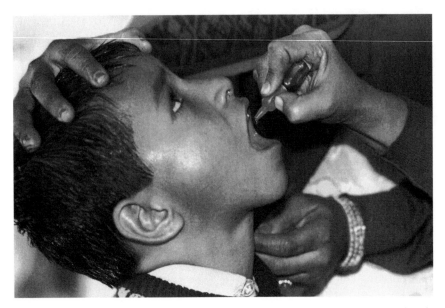

Ramesh Chander, aged 4, takes the oral polio vaccine at a health center in Mehurali village near New Dehli, India, on December 7, 1996. This was part of the campaign by the World Health Organization and Rotary International to eradicate polio world-wide. (AP Photo/Ajit Kumar)

countries. Europe, the Americas, and the Western Pacific regions containing half the world's population had all been certified polio free (Seytre and Shaffer, 2005, pp. 132–134). Even in countries where polio remained a problem, the disease had been eliminated from much of the country. In India, for example, polio cases were concentrated in the two poorest provinces, Uttar Pradesh and Bihar, and several provinces were polio free (Seytre and Shaffer, 2005, p. 129). There were also some setbacks. Several northern and heavily Muslim states in Nigeria suspended polio immunization because of suspicions that the vaccine was unsafe and might be sterilizing those who received it. As a result, the number of polio cases increased, and the disease spread to several neighboring countries. Eventually, polio vaccine manufactured in Indonesia, a Muslim country, reassured authorities in Nigeria and vaccination resumed. By 2008, the number of countries with endemic polio had been reduced to four: Afghanistan, India, Nigeria, and Pakistan. There were 1,486 polio cases in these endemic countries and another 132 cases in several other countries that were imported from one of the endemic countries (Global Polio Eradication Initiative, 2009, "Wild Polio Weekly Update"). Polio was proving more difficult to eradicate than smallpox.

As the campaign against polio moved into what doctors hoped was the end game, new challenges arose. As wild polio is eliminated, the only type of the poliovirus that circulates is that from the attenuated vaccine virus. Recent studies have suggested that the vaccine-derived virus can circulate in the community for many months following the last vaccination. And because it is a live, although weakened, virus, the vaccine-derived virus has shown some tendency to revert to a more virulent form capable of causing a case of paralytic polio. To prevent an epidemic of vaccine-derived poliovirus from occurring, medical authorities now know that they will have to maintain surveillance programs looking for polio-caused paralysis for some time following the elimination of wild polio. They will also have to maintain the capability to immunize populations at risk for a vaccine-derived poliovirus epidemic.

As of 2009, the goal of eradicating polio remains elusive. Substantial sums of money have been contributed to the campaign. Private organizations such as Rotary International, which has raised more than $700 million, and the Bill and Melinda Gates Foundation, which has contributed over $100 million, along with the World Health Organization, UNICEF, and many national governments have provided funding. In addition, millions of volunteers have made the national immunization days possible. The private fundraising and the extensive use of volunteers recall the successful efforts of the National Foundation for Infantile Paralysis and the March of Dimes to end the polio epidemics in the United States. Although the goal of eradicating polio has not yet been accomplished, the campaign against the disease in the last two decades has substantially reduced the number of children paralyzed and crippled by the disease.

CONCLUSION

Polio is an ailment whose emergence as an epidemic disease in the late nineteenth century was made possible by modernization and whose elimination as a major health threat in most of the world is the result of modern medical science. Polio would not have become epidemic without the development of modern sanitary practices that interrupted the continual circulation of the poliovirus in communities that exposed children to the virus at a young age when they had some protection from maternal antibodies. If modernization transformed polio from an endemic disease to an epidemic one of greater severity, it also spurred the scientific study of the disease. Developments in modern medical science, particularly in virology, eventually gave doctors the tools they needed to eliminate the threat of polio in much of the world by the early twenty-first century.

As we have seen, polio emerged as an epidemic disease in northern Europe and in the United States in the late nineteenth century as a result of improved sanitation. The scientific study of the disease and the poliovirus began in earnest in the early twentieth century following the discovery of the poliovirus by Karl Landsteiner. Simon Flexner and others in the United States soon took up the challenge of studying this newly emergent disease. These scientific studies were given new urgency following the massive 1916 polio epidemic in New York and the northeastern United States that sickened over 27,000 and killed over 8,000. But the poliovirus did not yield its secrets easily. In part, this was because Flexner and others primarily studied the disease in monkeys that they infected by giving them a shot of the virus in the nerves of the nose. But in humans, polio is typically acquired by ingesting the virus through the mouth, by which it moves into the intestines. By the late 1930s, doctors had begun to get a clearer picture of how polio was spread and what happened when the poliovirus infected an individual. Studies in the laboratory and in the field during polio epidemics eventually revealed the oral-fecal route of transmission, the fact that over 90 percent of all polio cases are inapparent, and the three different and independent strains of polio. In the late 1940s, John Enders, Thomas Weller, and Frederick Robbins discovered how to grow the poliovirus in non-nervous tissue, a necessary breakthrough for the development of any vaccine. Almost fifty years of research on the poliovirus and the disease bore fruit in the 1950s when Jonas Salk developed his inactivated polio vaccine and Albert Sabin created his attenuated live-virus vaccine. These two vaccines gave physicians the weapons they needed to significantly reduce the incidence of polio by the 1960s, particularly in the more developed nations of the world.

Polio also had significant cultural impact, particularly in the United States, which experienced some of the worst epidemics between 1916 and 1955. Most biographers and historians agree that his experience in dealing with polio helped shape Franklin D. Roosevelt's actions as one of the most important twentieth-century presidents. Roosevelt also helped transform the experience of having polio. By establishing the Warm Springs rehabilitation facility in Georgia in the late 1920s, Roosevelt helped demonstrate that polio victims could recover much of their function and resume their interrupted lives in spite of the disabilities. Roosevelt also lent his support to the establishment of the National Foundation for Infantile Paralysis (NFIP) under the leadership of his former law partner Basil O'Connor. The NFIP, and its fundraising arm the March of Dimes, raised millions of dollars to support polio patients' recovery and to fund most of the research that led to the successful vaccines. The NFIP also made polio the emblematic disease of mid-twentieth-century America. Its extensive campaigns to raise millions of dollars through small contributions, its public relations efforts to raise awareness of the disease and encourage contributions, and its widely disseminated warnings of the dangers of polio and advice about how to cope made polio into the most feared disease at mid-century.

The lives of the hundreds of thousands of polio survivors also had a significant cultural impact in the United States. Most emulated the example of Franklin Roosevelt in refusing to let polio restrict their possibilities. They underwent long and arduous rehabilitation so they could continue their education or return to work. They refused to be confined to institutions or the back bedrooms of their parents' houses and, instead, sought out an education to compensate for their physical limitations, found work, married, and had a family. Polio survivors were also at the forefront of the disability rights movement, beginning as early as the 1930s. They protested against discrimination and lobbied for legislative changes to guarantee their right to participate fully in American society. The United States is now a much more hospitable place for all disabled Americans—thanks in large part to the early and long-sustained efforts of polio survivors.

Polio has had a long history of infecting and crippling men, women, and children. For many centuries it was endemic, with the poliovirus always present, and it disabled many individuals every year. But in the long period of human history before the rise of modern medicine, polio was only one of many diseases that paralyzed bodies, and doctors did not identify it as a separate illness. The tools of modern medicine enabled doctors to identify the poliovirus as the causative agent of a disease that infected many but that paralyzed only a small portion of those infected. Those same tools have brought polio to the verge of eradication. Type II polio no longer circulates in the wild, and the numbers of individuals infected with Types I and II have been significantly reduced. As recently as 1988, polio infected over 350,000 individuals annually, while in recent years the total has been under 2,000 cases worldwide. With a lot of work and some luck, polio will soon be eliminated as a cause of misery and suffering in the world.

Polio Timeline

1580–1350 BC	Egyptian stele, or wall carving, illustrates a characteristic deformity of polio, suggesting polio is an ancient disease.
1600–1800	Scattered reports in medical writings of paralysis in children that could be describing cases of polio.
1772	Scottish novelist Sir Walter Scott has a probable case of polio at the age of eighteen months that leaves him with a lame leg.
1789	Dr. Michael Underwood, a London pediatrician, provides the first clinical description of poliomyelitis in his *Diseases of Children*.
1813	Italian physician and surgeon Giovanni Battista Monteggia gives a detailed description of polio in his *Instituzione Chirurgicale*.
1835	English physician John Badham describes four cases of sudden paralysis in children probably as the result of polio.

1840	The first detailed study of several polio cases is published by the German physician Jacob von Heine.
	Deformities possibly caused by possible polio cases in the Pittsburgh area are described by Dr. A. G. Walter.
1841	An apparent outbreak of polio in West Feliciana Parish, Louisiana, is described by Dr. George Colmer.
1870	Spinal cord lesions resulting from polio are first described in the medical literature by French doctors Jean-Martin Charcot and A. Joffroy.
1886	Dr. Mary Putnam Jacobi summarizes in a medical textbook the state of medical knowledge regarding polio. She introduces the term "infantile paralysis" to the United States.
1890	Swedish physician Karl Oskar Medin compiles a more complete clinical description of polio based on epidemics in Sweden.
1894	First sizeable polio epidemic (132 cases) in the United States occurs in Vermont and is described by Dr. Charles Caverly.
1905	Ivar Wickman, a Swedish physician, proposes to call the disease Heine-Medin disease. He also observes and describes the 1905 Scandinavian epidemic that had over 1,000 cases. He is the first to recognize the importance of abortive cases during an epidemic.
1907	Significant polio epidemic in New York of between 750 and 1,200 cases.
1908	Austrian scientists Karl Landsteiner and Erwin Popper demonstrate that polio is caused by a filterable virus.
1908–1912	Polio cases on the rise in the United States.
1909	Dr. Simon Flexner at the Rockefeller Institute in New York first isolates the poliovirus in the United States and initiates a research program on poliomyelitis.
1916	The northeastern United States, especially New York and New England, experience a devastating polio epidemic. There are over 27,000 cases and over 6,000 deaths in 26 states. New York City has 8,900 cases and 2,400 deaths.

| 1917 | Dr. George Draper publishes his study of polio, *Acute Poliomyelitis,* with solid information and some new ideas about the disease. Draper's book helps shape clinical understanding of the disease for two decades. |

1917   Dr. George Draper publishes his study of polio, *Acute Poliomyelitis,* with solid information and some new ideas about the disease. Draper's book helps shape clinical understanding of the disease for two decades.

1921   Franklin D. Roosevelt develops polio at the advanced age of 39.

1924   Roosevelt first visits the warm pools at Warm Springs, Georgia, in search of a cure for his paralysis.

1926   Roosevelt purchases the failing resort at Warm Springs, Georgia, with the intention of turning it into a polio rehabilitation facility. He also establishes the Georgia Warm Springs Foundation to provide funding for the facility.

1928   Roosevelt is elected governor of New York, and his law partner, Basil O'Connor, takes charge of the Georgia Warm Springs Foundation.

Roosevelt is elected governor of New York, and his law partner, Basil O'Connor, takes charge of the Georgia Warm Springs Foundation.

The tank respirator, or iron lung, is invented by Dr. Philip Drinker of the Harvard School of Public Health. It enables doctors to save polio patients whose breathing muscles are paralyzed.

1931   The Yale Poliomyelitis Unit is established at Yale University in response to a serious epidemic in New Haven, Connecticut. This group of doctors will perform significant clinical research into polio.

Drs. Frank M. Burnet and Jean Macnamara, two Australian researchers, demonstrate conclusively that there are at least two distinct strains of poliovirus.

1934   The first President's Birthday Ball celebrations are held around the United States to raise money for Warm Springs and for research into polio. The President's Birthday Ball Commission is established to administer and distribute the funds raised by the balls.

1935   Dr. Maurice Brodie and Dr. John Kolmer test their independently developed polio vaccines in humans. Both vaccines fail. Kolmer's vaccine causes numerous cases of polio and at least six deaths.

1938   The National Foundation for Infantile Paralysis (NFIP) is established, and Basil O'Connor becomes its director, a post he will hold until 1962. The NFIP will raise substantial sums of money to pay for polio rehabilitation, for research into the disease, and to train doctors, nurses, and therapists to treat it.

The comedian Eddie Cantor suggests calling the fundraising efforts of the NFIP the March of Dimes.

Dr. Thomas Rivers, a leading virologist, is appointed chairman of the NFIP's Committee on Scientific Research.

1940   Sister Elizabeth Kenny, an Australian nurse, arrives in the United States to demonstrate and advocate for her method of using hot wool packs to alleviate the pain of muscle contractures in acute polio and to advocate for her methods of polio rehabilitation.

1942   The Sister Kenny Institute is established in Minneapolis, Minnesota, to care for patients using Kenny's methods and to train other therapists in her methods of rehabilitation.

1947   Dr. Jonas Salk establishes his research laboratory at the University of Pittsburgh.

1948   Drs. John Enders, Thomas Weller, and Frederick Robbins succeed in growing poliovirus in non-nervous tissue. This is a crucial step toward the commercial production of a polio vaccine. The three doctors will win the Nobel Prize in Medicine in 1954 for this achievement.

1949   The NFIP establishes and funds the Polio Typing Program to establish the number of polio strains. By the time the program is completed in 1952, it establishes that there are only three distinct strains of polio in the world.

1951   Dr. Jonas Salk begins work on a killed-virus polio vaccine in his laboratory at the University of Pittsburgh.

Dr. Albert Sabin begins working on a live-virus vaccine in his laboratory at the University of Cincinnati.

1952   Dr. Jonas Salk begins testing his killed-virus polio vaccine in human volunteers at two institutions near Pittsburgh.

Dr. Dorothy Horstmann at Yale University and Dr. David Bodian at Johns Hopkins University establish that the poliovirus briefly circulates in a patient's blood before symptoms appear. This finding will be crucial to the development of a polio vaccine.

The United States experiences its worst polio year, with over 57,000 cases nationally.

1954   The national field trial of the Salk polio vaccine is directed by Dr. Thomas Francis of the University of Michigan. The trial involves over 1.3 million children whose parents had consented to participation.

1955   On April 12, Dr. Thomas Francis announces that the Salk vaccine is both safe and effective. It is licensed for use the same day by the U.S. government.

In April and May, over 200 polio cases occur among individuals vaccinated with the polio vaccine produced by the Cutter Laboratories. Eleven of those infected die. The Cutter Incident sets back polio vaccination, although vaccine from other laboratories is soon approved, and vaccine programs resume.

1958   The March of Dimes begins to consider moving beyond polio and to shift its focus to juvenile arthritis, birth defects, and prenatal care.

1959   Albert Sabin tests his attenuated live-virus polio vaccine in the Soviet Union. Some 10 million children are vaccinated in the trial.

1960   Albert Sabin conducts tests of his live-virus vaccine in the United States involving 200,000 individuals in the vicinity of Cincinnati.

1961   The American Medical Association recommends that the United States use the Sabin vaccine rather than the Salk vaccine.

The Sabin vaccine against Type I polio is licensed by the U.S. government.

1962	Sabin vaccines against Types II and III polio are licensed by the government. Sabin vaccines largely supplant the Salk vaccine in the United States.
1970–1980	Lameness surveys in the developing world reveal that polio continues to be a major cause of disability in much of the world outside of North America and Europe.
1985	The Pan American Health Organization (PAHO) begins an initiative to eradicate polio in North and South America by 1990.
1987	Rotary International, a worldwide service organization, starts a campaign to raise $120 million to eliminate polio in the world.
1988	The Rotary International Campaign against polio raises $247 million. The World Health Assembly resolves to eradicate polio by 2000. There are an estimated 350,000 polio cases in the world.
1991	The last case of wild polio in the Americas is diagnosed in Peru in September in a three-year-old boy, Luis Fermin Tenorio.
1992–1993	A polio epidemic in the Netherlands that begins in a group that refuses vaccination on religious grounds later spreads to Canada.
1994	North and South America are certified polio free by the International Commission for the Certification of Polio Eradication. China holds its first National Immunization Days and vaccinates 80 million children against polio.
1995	India holds its first National Immunization Days and vaccinates 87 million children against polio.
1996	The last case of wild polio is diagnosed in China. A large polio epidemic in Albania spreads to neighboring countries.
1997	The last case of wild polio in the Western Pacific region is diagnosed in Cambodia.

2000   The thirty-seven countries and territories in the Western Pacific region are certified to be polio free.

There are only 719 cases of wild polio worldwide, down from 350,000 in 1988.

2002   The European region of fifty-one countries is certified to be polio free. With the Americas and the Western Pacific regions also certified polio free, half of the world's population lives in areas where the threat of polio has been eliminated.

Polio is endemic in only seven countries in the world.

2003   Rotary International raises $119 million for the polio campaign, bringing its total to over $500 million.

Polio is endemic in only six countries (Nigeria, India, Pakistan, Niger, Afghanistan, and Egypt), down from 125 in 1988.

Vaccination is suspended in Nigeria because of concerns about the safety of the vaccine.

2004   Nigerian vaccination resumed.

2008   The Bill and Melinda Gates Foundation establish a challenge grant to Rotary to raise a total of $200 million to finish the eradication of polio.

Glossary

Abortive poliomyelitis: a case of polio in which the patient has no paralysis.

Acute poliomyelitis: the period following infection when the virus is active and the patient is sick with fever, headaches, muscle stiffness and weakness, and, in some cases, paralysis.

AIDS: Acquired Immune Deficiency Syndrome.

AMA: American Medical Association.

Anterior horn cells: the nerve cells in the back of the spinal cord that are damaged or destroyed by the poliovirus.

Antibodies: proteins in the body produced in response to infection by a virus; antibodies protect the body against a second infection by the same strain of the virus.

Autopsy: examination of a body following death to determine the cause of death.

Blood serum: the liquid left when the solids in blood, such as blood cells, are separated out.

Bulbar poliomyelitis: poliomyelitis in which the poliovirus has invaded the brainstem; can paralyze the muscles that control breathing and swallowing.

CDC: Communicable Disease Centers, now the Centers for Disease Control and Prevention.

Centers for independent living: centers where individuals with disabilities can receive assistance to live independently.

Chest respirators: a respirator to aid breathing that fits around the torso enabling a patient to sit and to be mobile.

Clinical pathology: study of disease processes in the body; the study of how the polio virus operates in the human body.

Clinical research: the study of disease processes in the human body.

Clinical virology: the study of how viruses operate in the body to create illnesses.

Controls: in a field trial of a vaccine or drug, those individuals who do not receive the vaccine or drug but who are observed to compare with those individuals who do receive the vaccine or drug.

Double-blind field trial: a field trial of a vaccine or drug in which neither the individual administering the vaccine or drug nor the patient knows whether the vaccine or drug is real or a placebo; used to eliminate possible bias in the results.

Epidemic disease: a disease that periodically infects all susceptible individuals in a community in a short period of time.

Endemic disease: a disease that is always present in a community.

Epidemiologist: a scientist who studies how disease spreads and the methods used to control spread.

Epidemiology: the study of how diseases are spread and controlled or prevented.

Fecal/oral route: the method by which the poliovirus enters the body; hands or food and water are contaminated by human waste and then taken into the mouth.

FDR: Franklin Delano Roosevelt.

Field trial: trial of a vaccine or drug to assess its safety and effectiveness in humans.

Filterable virus: a disease-causing organism small enough to slip through tiny holes in a laboratory filter that block larger organisms, such as bacteria, from going through.

Formalin: a preparation of the chemical formaldehyde used to kill or inactivate viruses for vaccines.

Frog breathing: using the throat muscles and tongue to force air into the lungs; used by polio patients whose breathing muscles were paralyzed; also known as glossopharyngeal breathing.

Glossopharyngeal breathing: using the throat muscles and tongue to force air into the lungs; used by polio patients whose breathing muscles were paralyzed; also known as frog breathing.

HEW: the Department of Health, Education, and Welfare in the United States government.

HIV: Human Immunodeficiency Virus; the cause of AIDS.

Hydrotherapy: use of warm water in a pool or tub to relax muscles and to facilitate physical therapy of weak or paralyzed muscles.

Immunization: using a vaccine to prevent infection by a virus or bacteria.

Inapparent poliomyelitis: poliomyelitis infection in which the individual exhibits no sign of illness; the vast majority of poliomyelitis infections were inapparent.

Incubation period: the period of time between when an individual is infected with a virus or bacteria and when he or she becomes sick.

Independent living movement: a movement to make it possible for individuals with disabilities to live independently by increasing accessibility.

Infantile paralysis: one of the names commonly used for poliomyelitis.

IPV: inactivated polio vaccine, such as the Salk vaccine.

Iron lung: tank respirator invented in 1928 and used to keep polio patients alive whose breathing muscles were paralyzed.

Isolation hospital/ward: a hospital or hospital ward used to isolate patients with contagious diseases such as polio.

Killed-virus vaccine: a vaccine in which the virus is killed but still capable of producing an antibody response, such as the Salk vaccine.

Live-virus vaccine: a vaccine in which the virus is weakened or attenuated but still capable of producing an antibody response but not the disease, such as the Sabin vaccine.

NFIP: National Foundation for Infantile Paralysis.

OPV: oral polio vaccine; a vaccine given by mouth, such as the Sabin vaccine.

Orthopedic surgeon: a surgeon who operates primarily on bones.

PAHO: Pan-American Health Organization.

Paralytic poliomyelitis: a case of poliomyelitis in which muscles are paralyzed.

Physical therapy: the use of exercises to restore strength to muscles weakened by disease or accident.

Physiotherapy: the use of exercises to restore strength to muscles weakened by disease or accident.

Placebo: an inactive substance used as a control in the field trial of a drug or vaccine.

Plague: a highly infectious disease that caused widespread death in the Middle Ages.

Poliomyelitis: an acute viral disease that in a small percentage of cases can cause muscle weakness or paralysis.

Polio pioneer: one of the children who participated in the 1954 field trial of the Salk vaccine.

Poliovirus: the virus that causes poliomyelitis.

Poster child: a child selected to represent a disease during a fundraising campaign.

Post-Polio Syndrome: a late effect of poliomyelitis in which individuals who had polio experience new pain, weakness, and fatigue several decades after their initial disease.

Protestant Work Ethic: a belief derived from Protestant theology that hard work pursued diligently over a long period will produce rewards.

Quarantine: enforced restrictions on individuals with a contagious disease.

Rocking beds: a bed that rocked like a teeter-totter; used to aid respiration in polio patients whose breathing muscles were weak or paralyzed.

Sabin vaccine: an oral, live-virus polio vaccine developed by Dr. Albert Sabin.

Salk vaccine: an injected, inactivated or killed-virus polio vaccine developed by Dr. Jonas Salk.

Scoliosis: an abnormal curvature of the spine caused in polio patients by weak or paralyzed muscles on one side of the torso.

Smallpox: an acute, epidemic viral disease that causes serious skin blisters; now thought to be eradicated as a result of vaccination

Spinal fusion: fusing the bones of the spine to correct or prevent scoliosis.

Spinal poliomyelitis: poliomyelitis in which the poliovirus damages or destroys the anterior horn cells of the spinal cord leading to muscle weakness or paralysis.

Spinal tap: using a long needle to take a sample of the fluid surrounding the spinal cord; used to diagnose poliomyelitis.

Tracheotomy: an operation that cuts a hole in the trachea, or windpipe, to insert a tube to assist breathing.

Typing program: a research program conducted to ascertain the number of strains of poliovirus circulating in the world.

UNICEF: United Nations Children's Fund, formerly United Nations International Children's Emergency Fund.

Vaccine: a prepared substance using either an inactivated or killed virus or bacteria that is capable of producing protective antibodies in humans.

Viremia: the presence of viruses or virus particles in the blood stream.

Virologist: a scientist who studies viruses.

Virology: the study of viruses.

Virus: a simple organism capable of causing illness; cannot reproduce except in an appropriate host.

Wards: large hospital rooms housing from four to twenty beds; common in hospitals in the mid-twentieth century.

WHO: World Health Organization.

Bibliography

Alexander, Larry, as told to Adam Barnett. 1954. *The Iron Cradle*. New York: Thomas Y. Crowell Company.

Benison, Saul. 1967. *Tom Rivers: Reflections on a Life in Medicine and Science*. Cambridge, MA: MIT Press.

Black, Kathryn. 1996. *In the Shadow of Polio: A Personal and Social History*. Reading, MA: Addison-Wesley Publishing Company.

Carter, Nancy Baldwin. 1998. "How I Learned to Make Peace with My Disability." In Lauro S. Halstead, ed. *Managing Post-Polio: A Guide to Living Well with Post-Polio Syndrome*. Washington, D. C.: NRH Press, pp. 220–224.

————. 2006. "Making Peace with My Aging Disability." In Lauro S. Halstead, ed. *Managing Post-Polio: A Guide to Living and Aging Well with Post-Polio Syndrome*, Second Edition. St. Petersburg, FL: ABI Professional Publications, pp. 215–221.

Carter, Richard. 1961. *The Gentle Legions*. Garden City, NY: Doubleday.

Chappell, Eleanor. 1960. *On the Shoulders of Giants: The Bea Wright Story*. Philadelphia: Chilton Company.

Daniel, Thomas M. 1997. "Polio and the Making of a Doctor." In Thomas M. Daniel and Frederick C. Robbins, eds. *Polio*. Rochester, NY: University of Rochester Press, pp. 79–96.

Davis, Fred. 1991. *Passage through Crisis: Polio Victims and Their Families*. New Brunswick, NJ: Transaction Publishers.

Doherty, Jim. 1997. "Chicago Changes." In *Memories: A Tribute to Polio Survivors*. Atlanta, GA: Atlanta Post-Polio Association, pp. 39–42.

Dunphy, Lynne M. 2001. "'The Steel Cocoon': Tales of the Nurses and Patients of the Iron Lung, 1929–1955." *Nursing History Review* 9: 3–33.

Eiben, Robert M. 1997. "The Polio Experience and the Twilight of the Contagious Disease Hospital." In Thomas M. Daniel and Frederick C. Robbins, eds. *Polio.* Rochester, NY: University of Rochester Press, pp. 97–119.

Emerson, Haven. 1917. *A Monograph on the Epidemic of Poliomyelitis (Infantile Paralysis) in New York City in 1916.* New York: Department of Health of New York City.

Finger, Anne. 2006. *Elegy for a Disease: A Personal and Cultural History of Polio.* New York: St. Martin's Press.

Gallagher, Hugh Gregory. 1998. *Black Bird Fly Away: Disabled in an Able-Bodied World.* Arlington, VA: Vandamere Press.

———. 1994. *FDR's Splendid Deception*, Revised Edition. Arlington, VA: Vandamere Press.

Global Polio Eradication Initiative. 2008. "The History." www.polioeradication.org/history.asp (accessed December 2008).

———. 2009. "Wild Poliovirus Weekly Update." www.polioeradication.org/history.asp (accessed January 2009).

Goldberg, Richard Thayer. 1981. *The Making of Franklin D. Roosevelt: Triumph over Disability.* Cambridge, MA: Abt Books.

Hall, Robert F. 1990. *Through the Storm: A Polio Story.* St. Cloud, MN: North Star Press of St. Cloud.

Historical Statistics of the United States, Colonial Times to 1970, Part I. 1975. Washington, D. C.: Government Printing Office.

"Incidence Rates of Poliomyelitis in the USA." 1999. *Polio Network News* 15: 3.

Kingery, Kenneth. 1966. *As I Live and Breathe.* New York: Grosset & Dunlap.

Kirkendall, Don, and Mary Phraner Warner. 1973. *Bottom High to the Crowd.* New York: Walker and Company.

Kriegel, Leonard. 1991. *Falling into Life.* San Francisco: North Point Press.

———. 1998. *Flying Solo: Reimagining Manhood, Courage, and Loss.* Boston: Beacon Press.

LeComte, Edward. 1957. *The Long Road Back: The Story of My Encounter with Polio.* Boston: Beacon Press.

Lewin, Philip. 1941. *Infantile Paralysis: Anterior Poliomyelitis.* Philadelphia: W. B. Saunders Company.

Little, Jan. 1996. *If It Weren't for the Honor—I'd Rather Have Walked: Previously Untold Tales of the Journey to the ADA.* Cambridge, MA: Brookline Books.

Marugg, Jim, and Anne Walters. 1954. *Beyond Endurance.* New York: Harper & Brothers Publishers.

Mee, Charles. 1999. *A Nearly Normal Life: A Memoir.* Boston: Little, Brown and Company.

Milam, Lorenzo W. 1984. *The Cripple Liberation Front Marching Band Blues.* San Diego, CA: Mho & Mho Works.

Needham, Jane Boyle, as told to Rosemary Taylor. 1959. *Looking Up.* New York: G. P. Putnam's Sons.

Nudelman, Dorothea, and David Willingham. 1994. *Healing the Blues: Drug-Free Psychotherapy for Depression.* Pacific Grove, CA: The Boxwood Press.

O'Brien, Mark, with Gillian Kendall. 2003. *How I Became a Human Being: A Disabled Man's Quest for Independence*. Madison: University of Wisconsin Press.

Offit, Paul A. 2005. *The Cutter Incident: How America's First Polio Vaccine Led to the Growing Vaccine Crisis*. New Haven, CT: Yale University Press.

Oshinsky, David M. 2005. *Polio: An American Story*. New York: Oxford University Press.

Paul, John R. 1971. *A History of Poliomyelitis*. New Haven, CT: Yale University Press.

Robbins, Frederick C. 1997. "Reminiscences of a Virologist." In Thomas M. Daniel and Frederick C. Robbins, eds. *Polio*. Rochester, NY: University of Rochester Press, pp. 121–134.

Rogers, Naomi. 1992. *Dirt and Disease: Polio before FDR*. New Brunswick, NJ: Rutgers University Press.

Rothman, David J. 1997. *Beginnings Count: The Technological Imperative in American Health Care*. A Twentieth Century Fund Book. New York: Oxford University Press.

Sass, Edmund J., George Gottfried, and Anthony Sorem. *Polio's Legacy: An Oral History*. Lanham, MD: University Press of America.

Seavey, Nina Gilden, Jane S. Smith, and Paul Wagner. 1998. *A Paralyzing Fear: The Triumph over Polio in America*. New York: TV Books.

Serotte, Brenda. 2006. *The Fortune Teller's Kiss*. Lincoln: University of Nebraska Press.

Seytre, Bernard, and Mary Shaffer. 2005. *The Death of a Disease: A History of the Eradication of Poliomyelitis*. New Brunswick, NJ: Rutgers University Press.

Shapiro, Joseph P. 1993. *No Pity: People with Disabilities Forging a New Civil Rights Movement*. New York: Times Books.

Sills, David L. 1957. *The Volunteers: Means and Ends in a National Organization*. Glencoe, IL: The Free Press.

Silver, Julie K. 2001. *Post-Polio: A Guide for Polio Survivors and Their Families*. New Haven, CT: Yale University Press.

Smith, Jane S. 1990. *Patenting the Sun: Polio and the Salk Vaccine*. New York: William Morrow.

Sternburg, Louis, Dorothy Sternburg, and Monica Dickens. 1986. *View from the Seesaw*. New York: Dodd, Mead, and Company.

Vastyshak, Kathryn. 2002. Interview with Daniel J. Wilson. Unpublished reference.

Ward, Geoffrey C. 1989. *A First-Class Temperament: The Emergence of Franklin Roosevelt*. New York: Harper & Row.

Wilson, Daniel J. 1998. "A Crippling Fear: Experiencing Polio in the Era of FDR." *Bulletin of the History of Medicine* 72: 464–495.

———. 2005. *Living with Polio: The Epidemic and Its Survivors*. Chicago: University of Chicago Press.

———. 2008 "Psychological Trauma and Its Treatment in the Polio Epidemics." *Bulletin of the History of Medicine* 82: 848–877.

Zola, Irving Kenneth. 1983. *Socio-Medical Inquiries: Recollections, Reflections, and Reconsiderations*. Philadelphia: Temple University Press.

Index

About the Author

DANIEL J. WILSON, Ph.D., has been teaching history of medicine for more than a decade and is professor of history at Muhlenberg College. He was a fellow with the Agency of Healthcare Research and Quality and The National Endowment for the Humanities. He has given presentations on the polio epidemics at meetings of the American Association for the History of Medicine, the American Historical Association, and the International Post-Polio and Independent Living Conference, as well as at Harvard University and Columbia University. Wilson is himself a polio survivor.